T0146662

Praise for **Cell-Level Healing**

"Science and spirit are brought together with beauty and discernment in this exquisite book. Joyce Hawkes offers us a vision of healing that truly manages to bridge worlds which only remain separate at our peril. 'The Bridge from Soul to Cell' is more than a good metaphor: it links wisdom and science and by doing so opens the way for great healing."

—**James O'Dea,** president, Institute of Noetic Sciences

"Joyce Hawkes blends and makes whole our splintered perceptions of the roles of science and spirit in healing. Her beautiful vision of how cells house the very power of the universe speaks to a greater understanding of the interconnectedness of the spiritual and the physical. In this broader understanding, Joyce bridges the gulf between the tangible and the intangible. She offers up the potential for self-healing, always waiting within us. Her book is both art and science for healing."

—**Joan C. King, PhD,** professor emerita, Tufts University School
of Medicine, and author of *Cellular Wisdom*

"The intrinsic nature of our being is primordially pure, luminous awareness—and mind and body are the unified expression of that reality. Dr. Hawkes's insightful work brings a depth of scientific knowledge together with the tools for applying that understanding in a way which relieves suffering and promotes spiritual awareness. *Cell-Level Healing* sheds welcome light on the interdependence of our inner and outer worlds. It provides practical guidance for working with the challenges of illness while supporting our journey of personal transformation."

—**Dzogchen Ponlop Rinpoche,** founder and president,
Nalandabodhi and Nitartha International,
and author of *Wild Awakening: The Heart of Mahamudra and Dzogchen*

"*Cell-Level Healing* is quite simply the whole exciting truth about how and why our consciousness is key to our physical health and well-being."

—**Christiane Northrup, MD,** author of *Mother-Daughter Wisdom, The Wisdom of Menopause,* and *Women's Bodies, Women's Wisdom*

"*Cell-Level Healing* is a remarkable book. It provides the reader with a poetic and visual text on self-healing and demonstrates how science and spirituality need not be opponents but can serve as allies in the reader's transformation. Dr. Joyce Hawkes has created a delightful user-friendly volume that can be read, savored, and re-read—one that is both simple and profound."

—**Stanley Krippner, PhD,** Saybrook Graduate School and Research Center, coeditor of *Varieties of Anomalous Experience,* and author of *Extraordinary Dreams and How to Work with Them*

Cell-Level Healing

Cell-Level Healing

The Bridge from Soul to Cell

Joyce Whiteley Hawkes, PhD

Foreword by Joan C. King, PhD

ATRIA PAPERBACK
New York London Toronto Sydney

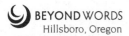
BEYOND WORDS
Hillsboro, Oregon

ATRIA PAPERBACK
A Division of Simon & Schuster, Inc.
1230 Avenue of the Americas
New York, NY 10020

BEYOND WORDS
20827 N.W. Cornell Road, Suite 500
Hillsboro, Oregon 97124-9808
tel: 503-531-8700   fax: 503-531-8773
www.beyondword.com

The information contained in this book is intended to be educational and not for diagnosis, prescription, or treatment of any health disorder whatsoever. This information should not replace consultation with a competent healthcare professional. The content of the book is intended to be used as an adjunct to a rational and responsible healthcare program prescribed by a professional healthcare practitioner. The author and publisher are in no way liable for any misuse of the material.

Managing editors: Henry Covey, Lindsay S. Brown
Editor: Teresa Barker
Proofreaders: Jessica Bryan and Marvin Moore
Design: Carol Sibley, Devon Smith
Composition: William H. Brunson Typography Services

First Atria Paperback/Beyond Words trade paperback edition June 2011

ATRIA PAPERBACK and colophon are trademarks of Simon & Schuster, Inc.
Beyond Words Publishing is a division of Simon & Schuster, Inc.

For more information about special discounts for bulk purchases, please contact Simon & Schuster Special Sales at 1-866-506-1949 or business@simonandschuster.com.

The Simon & Schuster Speakers Bureau can bring authors to your live event. For more information or to book an event, contact the Simon & Schuster Speakers Bureau at 1-866-248-3049 or visit our website at www.simonspeakers.com.

Manufactured in the United States of America

10 9 8 7 6 5 4 3 2

The Library of Congress has cataloged the hardcover edition as follows:

Hawkes, Joyce Whiteley.
      Cell-level healing : the bridge from soul to cell / Joyce Whiteley Hawkes. — 1st ed.
         p. cm.
      1. Energy--Therapeutic use. 2. Vital force--Therapeutic use. 3. Mind and body therapies. 4. Self-care, Health. I. Title.
      RZ421.H39   2006
      615.8'52—dc22

                                                                              2006018855

ISBN: 978-1-58270-146-2 (hc)
ISBN: 978-1-58270-313-8 (pbk)
ISBN: 978-1-4516-2901-9 (eBook)

The corporate mission of Beyond Words Publishing, Inc.: *Inspire to Integrity*

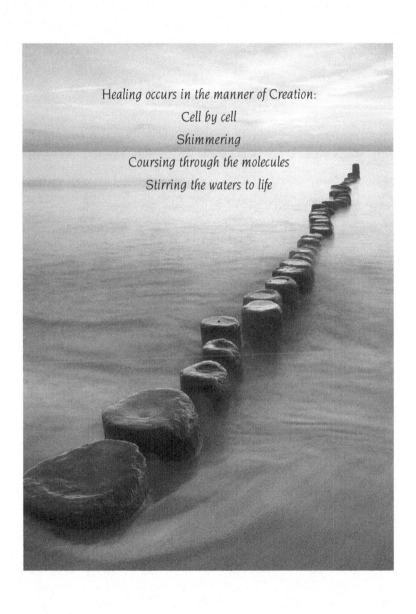

Healing occurs in the manner of Creation:

Cell by cell

Shimmering

Coursing through the molecules

Stirring the waters to life

Contents

Contents

Foreword

History is rich with humans going beyond defined barriers. Acts of bravery, discoveries in science, messages of hope and peace, and initiations into the deeper mysteries of who we are forever change our human paradigm. These souls have journeyed beyond and back again.

Poet Theodore Roethke wrote, "I learn by going where I have to go," and I would add, "We teach what we need to learn." Both these phrases describe Dr. Joyce Whiteley Hawkes's journey to her present life's work as a biophysicist who answered the call to healing after her own near-death experience. Engaged in healing now for more than twenty years, she blends and makes whole our splintered perceptions of science and spirit in healing by bridging the tangible cell with the intangible spirit.

Meeting Joyce seven years ago, I immediately recognized the power of her deep knowledge of cells infused with her direct experience of healing. In *Cell-Level Healing*, she presents us with a greater understanding of the interconnectedness of the spiritual and the physical. Her story intertwines these two realms in her unique vision of cells—powerhouses of the universe—and offers us concrete principles and step-by-step road maps and exercises, together with beautiful images, to promote self-healing.

Foreword

Beyond her descriptive understanding of the process of healing, beyond thoughts of wellness, her words challenge our mind's understanding about the nature of reality, time, and space. We are both *in* and *of* the process of rejuvenating the physical through spirit.

Our compassionate hearts swell with possibilities to reach out and partake in the restoration of our selves and others. Our touch becomes sacred. We are here, standing on the bridge between Soul and Cell, embracing both with new awareness thanks to Joyce and what she has learned on her journey.

Travel with her now in a quantum leap beyond the physical cell to the spiritual, housed in the words of this book. Dr. Hawkes can guide you there, toward the dawn of your own renaissance of health.

Cell-Level Healing asks us to revisit our bodies from a position of the sacred, journey deep into the mystery of our own human potential; and contemplate the power of the universe convening in our cells.

—Joan C. King, Ph.D., professor emerita, Tufts University School of Medicine, and author of *Cellular Wisdom*

Acknowledgments

**Many of my friends and clients
have encouraged, cajoled, and inspired this book.
I thank them all, with all my heart, and in particular I wish to thank:**

Teresa Barker, whose encouragement kept me going, and whose editorial comments have significantly improved this work.

Marilyn Rossner, Ph.D., of Montreal, who cheered me on more than once.

Marian Svinth, Ph.D., and Gene Slape, dear friends, whose encouragement and skills kept either the computer or me working.

Chris Standage, Mike Buckley, Dan Trythall, Joyce Izumi, Martha Blomberg, Joyce Liechenstein, Ph.D., Fadel Behman, Ph.D., Sally O'Neil, Ph.D., Hetty Kouw, Robert Schore, M.D., D. J. Zentner, Kim Clark Sharp, Melvin Morse, M.D., Sandy Woodward, Carla Stehr, and Toni Diane Holm, who all contributed in many ways.

My dearest daughter, Annalisa, for her life, joy, and love.

The Divine Source, who created mountains—like Mount Baker—for inspiration and play, and who placed within all of us the yearnings, designs, and bridges for health.

Last, but certainly not least, thanks to the staff at Beyond Words Publishing, Inc., for their consummate skill and integrity as publishers.

Introduction

**The tools for healing
presented in this book are
simple, powerful, and available to everyone.**
They reside within you, created as part of your genetic code, and they are a natural property of the intrinsic workings of every cell in your body. Appreciation of the gift of a body is the first step toward unlocking the spiritual energy available to assist you in your life journey. You can clear blockages, promote the flow of energy throughout your body, and apply cellular knowledge to specific situations and illnesses. These tools are time-tested, adaptable, and ready to be used for personal transformation. Deep healing is always available in present time. It can also reach back in time to heal past wounds.

There is a bridge between ordinary reality and spiritual reality that provides access to luminous meditation, healing energy, and wisdom. This bridge reaches directly into the units of life in the physical body: the cells. The energy of healing can touch and positively affect the inner workings of the cells where the information, action, power, and communication of the body does the work of life.

*There is a bridge between ordinary reality
and spiritual reality.*

Introduction

This book provides step-by-step instructions to help people find their own way of linking Soul to Cells. The chapters are organized to guide you through the Cell-Level Healing experience. Chapters 1 through 5 focus on initial preparation:

- Body awareness that leads to gratitude, compassion, and healing

- The means to identify and clear blockages

- The Principle of Flow, essential to Cell-Level Healing

Chapter 6 takes us inside the cells, where you'll see how nearly every cell in your body has the capability for

- Information

- Action

- Power

- Communication

Chapters 7 and 8 apply Cell-Level Healing to specific conditions and situations. Actual stories about individual healings, drawn from the author's twenty years in private practice, offer examples of how to navigate the Bridge from Soul to Cell.

In the center of this book, beginning on page 47, you'll find a section of photographs and other illustrations titled "Your Bridge from Soul to Cell."

A step-by-step guide, this section will help you to quiet your mind and connect with your inner energy for renewal by means of imagery that I have specifically chosen for this purpose. Exercises

Introduction

and meditations accompany the vivid photos of cells and those of other beautiful aspects of nature and invite you to enter your own healing practice. My hope is that you will tuck this book in a pocket, backpack, or purse and return to this healing portfolio again and again, discovering each time a new facet of the Cell to Soul healing experience.

In the journey toward total freedom, this book will empower you by placing the skills necessary for healing into *your own hands*. You will learn how to explore paths to health and joy far beyond your present imagination. Bridges to healing stretch from our souls to our emotions and through our minds to the teaming mass of our cells, bringing peace and vitality, joy and health.

Allow the words on the following pages to gently filter through your mind and assist you in beginning your Cell-Level Healing.

How a Scientist Became a Healer

**In my wildest dreams
I could not imagine falling in love with a cell,
but that happened the first time I looked into an electron microscope.**
There it was: a cell, gloriously magnified tens of thousands of times, showing each intricate detail of its unimaginably exquisite interior. Under the electron beam, there was no place for the cell to hide, and it graciously revealed some of its secrets. I loved the inside view, the images that could be seen only with the help of advanced scientific instrumentation.

This book is about cells and their relationship to energy healing, as experienced from my perspective as a scientist grounded in traditional cell research and as a healer who is attuned to the power of cells for repair and renewal. For nearly fifteen years—before the event that would shatter my view of reality—I studied and published scientific papers. My research looked at how cells become ill and how they survive, or not.

This book is about cells and their relationship to energy healing.

Early in my career, my passion was science. I completed my doctoral work at Pennsylvania State University in 1971 with a Ph.D.

in biophysics. Moving to Oregon, my postdoctoral position with the National Institutes of Health took me to a regional Primate Research Center. Soon I was publishing and speaking at conferences from New York to Seattle, where I eventually set up an electron microscope research facility for the National Marine Fisheries Service. This was a busy and productive laboratory, as I had five research assistants and graduate students and was an adjunct professor in the Department of Zoology at the University of Washington. My life involved traveling nationally and internationally, lecturing, publishing, and spending hours peering into an electron microscope to record the struggles of cells that had been poisoned by pollutants, such as PCBs and oil slicks. I published fifty scientific documents and was honored with a U.S. Department of Commerce National Achievement Award. Another highlight of my career was election to the position of Fellow in the American Association for the Advancement of Science, an ongoing position that I hold presently.

My research depended on the sophisticated technology of the electron microscope to illuminate the ultrasmall world inside of cells. This type of microscope is as big as a baby elephant and weighs about one ton. Multiple steps are required to "fire up" the microscope, which pours 100,000 volts of electricity through a filament that showers electrons down a series of electromagnetic lenses. Magnified up to a million times, the images revealed my passion: the inner workings of cells. Still, something beckoned me beyond all my accomplishments as a scientist.

The components of cells are not unique to humans. In fact, the parts of our cells are indistinguishable from those of all other living creatures. However, our genetic code, contained in the molecules of

How a Scientist Became a Healer

DNA in each cell, is as different from other species as we are from each other. These individual, personal codes create each unique body shape and individual characteristic. All this finely orchestrated complexity comes from one single fertilized egg cell holding half of our DNA from our mother and half from our father's sperm. Page 50 shows a sperm and egg at the moment before the amazing act of conception unites them as one, original cell, beginning the life of an individual organism.

As a scientist, I was dedicated to the pursuit of truth through scientific means. Religion and God were not part of my beliefs. Imagine my surprise one day when a decorative leaded-glass window fell off a mantel onto my head, initiating a classic near-death experience (often referred to as a "NDE"). I had never heard about the near-death experience, let alone been someone to whom out-of-the-ordinary or unexplainable things happened. I remember the oak-framed glass falling toward me and the crushing moment of impact.

Suddenly reality shifted, and I was no longer confined to my crumpled body collapsed on the floor. Instead, I was speeding down a long, dark tunnel, drawn to an incredible light in the distance. Without conscious control over the situation, a force outside myself stopped me at the entrance to the light. There, my mother and grandmother, long departed from this earth, greeted me. Overwhelmed with love and recognition, and amazed at their health and happiness, I was drawn past them over a threshold and into a whole other world.

Suddenly reality shifted, and I was no longer confined to my crumpled body collapsed on the floor.

Cell-Level Healing

No people or beings appeared. Rolling hills, the greenest grass, and colorful flowers glowed with light, seemingly from within each blade and petal. Colors appeared almost alive in their vividness. Utter clarity of image and hue surrounded me in all directions. Immersed in light and tranquillity, I soaked up these dazzling images and feelings, content to dwell forever in that place. Then the experience changed.

I was shifted instantaneously to standing in front of a Great Light. The overwhelming love and peace I had felt before this moment was only a minuscule taste of what emanated from the Light. The form was somewhat taller than a person, with the shape of a person but without distinct features. Everything and nothing seemed to exist simultaneously in this luminosity. I felt utterly blissful, alert, and full of love and joy. If this was God who greeted me, there was no judgment issued. I was totally loved, surrounded by peace and safety, and healed of everything that had ever caused disease or discomfort. The ecstasy of the moment suspended and transcended all time and space. It would later prove to be a bridge that I could access in order to return to this state of being at will.

There was no discussion about returning to Earth and no instructions were given. Just as suddenly as everything else had happened, I was thrust back into normal consciousness on the floor in my house—with a very sore head, a gash of fair proportions, and dried blood matted in my hair. Thus began my journey from my work as a scientist to my new calling as a Cell-Level Healer.

At first, my scientist's brain discounted the experience as a hallucination, merely the consequence of a sound crack on the head and loss of consciousness. But, I soon discovered, it was the beginning of another form of consciousness that would prove to be more valuable than any career, status, or fringe benefits.

My head hurt too much to listen to music, read, go to the movies, or exercise—all of the forms of relaxation I had previously enjoyed. Trapped in a fit body with a sorely pounding head and a physician-imposed three weeks at home, I was utterly bored. When I had recovered enough to drive, I went downtown to Seattle's waterfront area to visit my favorite bookstore, Elliot Bay Books. Creaking wooden floors and the aroma from decades of books comforted my senses.

I was walking slowly along the rows of shelves, browsing the titles, when a book nearly jumped into my hands. It was Ray Moody's *Life After Life: The Investigation of a Phenomenon—Survival of Bodily Death*, and it contained page after page of detailed near-death experiences.[1] I purchased the book, and reading it forced me to look closely at the evidence presented by the many others who had experiences similar to mine. I could no longer dismiss what had happened to me. Wonder and curiosity began replacing my grouchy self-pity at having a wounded skull.

Another man named Ray, a podiatrist, showed up in my life. Trained by the Super Learning group at Ohio State University, Ray taught memory skills via deep relaxation and visualization techniques. Don't ask what this had to do with feet! Seemingly unrelated to my recent experience, I embarked on memory training to help keep authors and citations straight in my work as a publishing scientist.

1. Raymond Moody, *Life After Life: The Investigation of a Phenomenon—Survival of Bodily Death*, 2nd ed. (San Francisco: HarperSanFrancisco, 2001).

Cell-Level Healing

In our session one day, I reclined in a big, comfortable chair in Ray's office, listening to a tape describing in detail the features of a small, gray kitten. I was a little surprised when, in my mind's eye, I saw myself walking around a room looking at specific things: a chair with blue velvet upholstery, a fireplace that was open on two sides into the room, and pictures on the wall. Even more surprising was the look on Ray's face when I described the room. We were both astonished when I described with precise detail the setting in which he had produced the memory tape. Put two scientists together and you launch a truth-seeking mission. We decided to discover how my inner sight worked in a real-time situation. I would go to Ray's office and relax in the big chair, and after we had chatted for a while, Ray would go down the hall and examine one of his podiatry patients. When he returned, I could tell him details about the person's foot, the pathology, and anything else that had caught his attention during the examination.

Put two scientists together and you launch
a truth-seeking mission.

We also established an informal mini-study in mind reading. Ray would think about a particular color as he walked to the room where I was waiting, and my head would be filled with that exact color. I was not guessing; I saw the color accurately every time. My view of myself as a levelheaded, rational scientist became unhinged. Perhaps you, too, have had some unusual experiences that scared you, at first, and then opened you to far-reaching possibilities in your life.

I began to look for information about other strange phenomena, such as the sixth sense, inner sight, and remote viewing. I joined a class given by a local healer. The meditations in class helped me establish a deep meditative practice at home, which led to visionary encounters with angels, animals, and other galaxies.

The teacher invited me to accompany him during his work with clients one afternoon a week, and people began responding positively to my touch. They told me they felt heat in the areas where I had touched them and that tingling shot through their body. They said their health improved as a result.

Others wanted to come to me for healing sessions, so I converted a former study in my home into a place where I could see a few clients each week. Never imagining anything but an avocation of heart, I enjoyed both worlds: science and whatever this new arena might be.

I continued to be challenged to reach deeper and deeper into the cells of the body in order to assist those who sought my help. The results astonished both my clients and myself.

During a long weekend trip to Mount Shasta with my teacher and two other students, my life changed precipitously, once again. We climbed to Red Butte from Panther Meadows on the south side of the mountain. Still snowy, the spring days were enchanting as we chopped steps in icy slopes, heated pots of snow to melt for drinking water, and settled into intensely blissful meditations at the 9,600-foot elevation.

On the drive back to Seattle, we four grubby pilgrims stopped at a Catholic shrine, the Grotto, on the outskirts of Portland, Oregon. I had no previous exposure to the Catholic church or theology, having grown up mildly Protestant. My companions went to pray in a small chapel, while I wandered alone and eventually stood in front of a room-sized cave that had been naturally formed in the side of a steep cliff. Candles flickered around a replica statue of the Pieta. Mary seemed almost alive as she sorrowed over the crucified body of Jesus.

As I approached the cave and knelt on a bench provided for worship, I felt the air shift and become charged with power and energy. I felt a tingling all over my body when I heard a woman's voice say, "You are called to heal."

It felt like the near-death experience all over again. Love, peace, and awe surged through me. How could I contain this emotion, this energy, this blessing? My life changed forever in those few moments. The loving authority in the voice left no room for doubt or delayed action. When I returned to Seattle and work the very next day, I began my resignation process to leave the laboratory.

The world of healing did not come naturally. I could not "think" my way to solutions as I had with science. I meditated regularly, sought divine guidance, and received it every step of the way, usually no sooner than the instant it was needed. My path evolved daily in the healing room and took quantum leaps during time spent with indigenous healers in Southeast Asia. Now, after twenty years of learning how to reach deeply into the cells of the body with healing energy, I am eager to share the wonder of weaving together the spirit world and physical healing.

My near-death experience established a connection between me and something much, much bigger than myself. If it is a part of God, the Source of Creation, the bond has never failed. I lost my fear of death, and with it, my fear of separation from the Source. I lost any notion that the Source is available to only the few who belong to a specific religion. The Healing Presence of the Source is for everyone.

How a Scientist Became a Healer

So, what about those cells? Is there love after the laboratory? Certainly the cells mean even more to me now. After all, physical health begins in our cells. Likewise, healing *must* touch the cells, because illness also begins at the cellular level.

Healing must touch the cells, because illness begins at the cellular level.

Did you know that individual cells seldom get completely sick all at once? Simple practices can help you support injured cells on the road to recovery. For example, Jerry, one of my first clients, was a construction worker with a new diagnosis of multiple sclerosis (MS). He had lost most of the strength in his dominant hand and could no longer wield a hammer or steady a nail driver. The vision in his right eye was blurred from time to time, and the unreliability of simple physical functions, such as sight and arm strength, frustrated him. We began healing work together, and within two weeks his vision was normal. Several months later, Jerry arrived at my office carrying a heavy jug of water in his right hand. He thrust it into my face with a huge grin of delight. Three months earlier, he had not been able to hold an orange in that hand. Both his eyes and the nerve cells in his body had healed.

The more you know about your body—and the cells of your body—the more you will appreciate how truly precious and sacred all life is. Rather than struggle against the body and our sojourn here on earth, the body can be experienced as a sacred temple of the spirit and an expression of consciousness. This knowledge is the first step toward a life of fullness and oneness of spirit and physical existence—a seamless connection from Soul to Cell.

2

The Heart of It All

**During the first years after the intensity of being
"on the other side," as I call my near-death experience,
I wanted to return to that place where there was only peace and love.**
I wondered why I was given a taste of heaven and then dumped back
into the dense physical world.

I asked for guidance: "Show me what this means. Show me!" To
receive answers required a change in my meditation practice. Rather
than journeying as far from my body as my imagination, drumming,
or the scent of roses could take me, I concentrated on staying with my
physical body. Instead of leaving the body, I tugged at my higher consciousness, bringing it forth, bit by bit, from deep within. I began to
feel a bit of heaven right here. From this, I developed a two-step practice that helps me connect with my higher consciousness in daily life.

*Gratitude leads to devotion, resulting in
compassion that flows naturally from the
heart as profound healing.*

Step One

Begin with the practice of appreciation, which can open you to receive
good things. Gratitude leads to devotion, resulting in compassion

that flows naturally from the heart as profound healing. An attempt to heal your body, or to help someone else heal, makes no sense if you lack respect and appreciation for your physical body and the physical universe. Fulfilling your heart's desire and your soul's mission requires presence in the here and now, and that includes awareness of your body.

The human body is amazing and deserves honest appreciation. The sheer number of cells in your body, nearly 100 trillion, outnumbers the entire population of the earth by 1,500 times and the stars of the Orion Galaxy by 1,000. Cells belong to *action groups*, or tissues, each with their own shape, size, job, and rate of cell division for renewal and repair of wornout parts. These trillions of cells work together to keep you alive.

Let appreciation fill and warm your body. Invite more of your higher consciousness, your spirit, to emerge from within you. Contemplate yourself in a new way using a special phrase, such as "at one with the Universe," "resting in luminosity," or "in the temple of the Holy Spirit."

BRIDGE TO HEALING

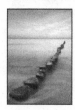 Take a moment to focus on four attributes you appreciate about your body. Record your thoughts in a personal journal for further reflection.

Step Two

The breath is a potent meditation tool in many traditions. Use it to expand your awareness of the higher aspects of yourself. Sometimes the sense of self, or soul, seems far away, as if needing retrieval. Invite all parts of your true self to come home to your heart.

BRIDGE TO HEALING

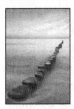 Let your breath expand your chest as you become filled with your own spirit. Visualize your entire being expanding and filling with the qualities of higher consciousness. Allow yourself to be infused with wisdom and compassion for yourself and all other beings. From its enormous expanse to its tiniest known particle, the universe is infused with luminous energy and wisdom. The four primary attributes of the cosmos can help us work with our most basic nature for healing: mystery, creativity, dynamic balance of flow and organization, and resilience.

Mystery

Huge parts of the universe can be seen, but even more remain hidden. The latest estimate is that we can perceive 4 percent of matter and energy, and this is only because some form of light is reflected or emitted by those parts. A whopping 96 percent of the universe is beyond our view because it is not in the visible spectrum. It is undetectable matter.[1] Likewise, the universe is known in some small portion by nearly all of us, but we continue to search for

1. Charles Seife, "Breakthrough of the Year: Illuminating the Dark Universe," *Science* 302 (2003): 2038; Seife, "What is the Universe Made Of?" *Science* 309 (2005): 5731.

answers to the great mysteries. How much is unknown? Who can estimate the immensity of discovery awaiting us? How much phenomenal energy is available for healing?

Creativity

The universe continually creates itself. In the tiny world of the proton, the positive center of each atom, a cauldron of creation stirs in each fraction of a second. Just like outer space, once thought to be a vacuum of total nothingness, the inner space of the proton actually holds huge amounts of energy. Every *nanosecond*—a time so small that more than a million nano-events occur in one blink of your eyelid—"something" forms out of the energy within the proton. One of these "somethings" is called a *gluon*. Known for their ability to hold the substance of the world together, gluons flash and then disappear. Gluons are only one of the many things that have spin and charge but no matter. They exist in protons for brief moments of time.

The universe continually creates itself.

Think about the trillions of cells in your body, recalling that you have more cells in your single body than the entire population of the earth. It's mind-boggling to imagine the number of molecules making up the cells. Then add to that the trillions and trillions of atoms making up the molecules.

There is an energy source that is constantly creating and dissolving gluons at the heart of each atom. Therefore, the flux of new creation is one of the deepest patterns within you. Each human being naturally possesses an astronomical amount of energy for new life and renewed health.

The Heart of It All

Dynamic Balance

The cosmos is constantly in flux as it creates new stars and recycles old ones. The universe balances creation and destruction in an orderly and elegant manner. It is no longer thought of as a giant clock wound tight at the beginning of time and left to run down into nothing.

The human body is a flowing system that continually balances input and output. Neither rigidly controlled nor left to the whims of chance, healthy systems are beautifully organized and fluidly balanced. This structure supports adaptability and stability at the same time. For example, muscle has a very ordered fiber composition that enables it to carry out both smooth and complex movement.

The universe balances creation and destruction in an orderly and elegant manner.

Nerves tell the muscles to move. Take, for example, what happens when you want to move your leg. A signal from the central nervous system is sent through the nerves to the leg muscles where the tiny fibers of two proteins, *actin* and *myosin*, slide together, contracting the muscles, lifting the thigh, and thereby raising your foot. In order to lower the foot back to the ground, they slide apart, relaxing the muscle.

Biochemistry aids in accessing nutrients and enables the complexity of movement. These miracles are too often taken for granted. Imagine trying to think your way through every minuscule event in order to take even one step. Then consider how many steps you take each day.

Cell-Level Healing

Regardless of how out-of-balance your body may have become, it still retains the information necessary to return to balance. Learning to restore peaceful, healthy balance is just one gift of the bridge to healing.

Regardless of how out-of-balance your body may have become, it still retains the information necessary to return to balance.

Resilience

Ages ago, our ancestors looked at the stars and noticed that the same constellations appeared season after season. Rotating with a predictable pattern, the idea of a clock with planets and stars going around and around made logical sense. The black space in which the stars moved looked empty and therefore became known as just that: empty.

How different our current views are! We now know that empty space is vibrant with energy and the heavens are not fixed. New stars form all the time, old ones explode, and black holes gobble up and smash together any matter daring to come close to them. Immensely resilient in resources, the universe constantly renews and repairs itself.

Our bodies reflect this same quality of resilience. Minor injuries merely slow us down. Cut your finger and a complex series of steps is initiated to stop the bleeding, seal off the wound, and form a mat of fibers for new cells to use as a matrix during repair. When the repair is complete, the fibers dissolve. If the wound is too large, a visible scar will form to close the area and protect the integrity of the inner layers.

The Heart of It All

During times of major healing crises, the natural resilience of the body can be affirmed in order to shorten the time needed for healing and encourage our spirits as we move through the process.

BRIDGE TO HEALING

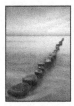

Write in your journal or simply go to page 62 to reflect about how you personally embody the four primary attributes of the cosmos in your body and in your life: mystery, creativity, dynamic balance of flow and organization, and resilience. Your perception of this may change from day to day. You may enjoy repeating this exercise frequently as a basis for meditation.

3

Clearing Blockages

**Early in my healing practice,
I thought my job was to meditate, fill myself with
healing energy, and blast my client with it—to the best of my ability.**
On rare occasions, the outcome dazzled: sudden reversals of arthritis, shriveled cancers. More often than not, the results did not reflect the endeavor. Some clients even became nauseated.

Puzzled by these inconsistent results, I sought answers. I discovered that people who had already done a considerable amount of spiritual or meditative practice were able to receive and utilize a substantial flow of energy. Those who were just starting to meditate and awaken spiritually, or who were just beginning some other form of complementary healing, had the most difficulty. Seeking the advice of a wise Chinese physician and acupuncturist, I learned about the concept of *blockage*, which is so thoroughly understood in his tradition. Energy blockage prevents healing, no matter how much energy is available. This new awareness helped me to understand the variable results I was seeing in my healing practice.

*Energy blockage prevents healing, no matter
how much energy is available.*

I realized that in addition to sharing healing energy with my clients, I needed to find out more specifically where the energy blockages were and clear them. The more specifically I could locate them, the better the healing.

I began using a pendulum, which would begin to spin when I held it above the blocked area. I found this method to be generally reliable. Soon, I was able to sense the blocked places with my hands. A cold wind or excess heat would come from the sites of disease or former injury. Sometimes, I could see the blockage with my eyes, or I might have an uncanny sense of *knowing* where the problem originated.

Not all blockages are easy to clear. Energy obstructions can be especially tenacious when a belief system has locked them into place. Jocelyn's case illustrates a limiting belief system that obstructed her from healing. Her case is not unusual. I have heard hundreds of similar stories.

• • •

Tears poured down Jocelyn's face as she walked from my reception area into the office. She slumped onto the comfy couch, clutched the sky-blue chenille decorative cushion, and launched immediately into her concerns.

"I was diagnosed with breast cancer a month ago, and I had surgery three weeks ago. The doctor found a very aggressive tumor. I'm scheduled to start chemotherapy the end of this week. I read that I need to find the cause of the cancer before I can heal.

"I don't know where to look. My brother abused me when I was sixteen. I was terribly mean to my kid sister after that. Am I being punished? What did I do to cause my cancer?"

Clearing Blockages

• • •

Certainly many factors can contribute to illness, including emotional trauma, genetic predisposition, and environmental toxic exposure. We tend to extrapolate backwards, however, from the disease to a simplistic cause, particularly one that points the finger of blame toward others or guilt toward ourselves.

Jocelyn's generally intense emotions and all-consuming guilty thoughts contributed to her state of phenomenal stress. The serious effects of stress include depression of the immune system and reduced nerve regeneration (*neurogenesis*), both of which can block the healing of the body.

Although the cause of Jocelyn's cancer was unknown, her stress clearly undermined her well-being and blocked her recovery. Confused and upset by surgery, chemotherapy, and other treatments, it took all her courage just to face each day. We needed to help her find tools to reduce her stress. We used imagery of Jocelyn walking along her favorite stretch of beach listening to the crashing waves, smelling the fresh salt air, and feeling the warmth of sun on her shoulders. We continued using imagery that she could initiate and change whenever she needed to make the process uniquely her own. She not only found peace of mind but eventually resolved her feelings of guilt and let go of her suspicion that she was being taught a lesson for having done something wrong.

Months after she had completed her course of medical treatment—and her formerly bald head sported a vigorous cap of new, fuzzy growth—we looked back on the intrusion of cancer and what she learned from the experience.

"I have new insights about my life," she said. "I'm a good person with gifts that help others. I count to a lot of people. All the 'things' I've accumulated mean much less to me now. Material possessions are no longer an important goal. My priorities have changed, and I am happy and free to enjoy my life and my loved ones. With your help, I was able to focus on using healing meditations in conjunction with the best possible medical treatment, and I was able to get through my cancer."

Jocelyn's main blockage was the belief that her illness was punishment. Once she was able to clear this limitation, her body responded. She had fewer aftereffects from chemotherapy, less fatigue, and a much increased sense of well-being. Her confidence that she actually had a good future increased, too. The outcome of her illness included physical healing plus a new level of wisdom about herself and her life. Beliefs are powerful tools that can limit us, but they can also be used to propel us into life-giving freedom.

Limiting beliefs obstruct emotional, physical, and spiritual healing, but the energy that holds obstructions can be released. The information in the rest of this chapter can help you learn to locate blockages. Tools for release are also included.

Clearing Emotional Blockages

Decades ago, veterans returned from Vietnam with severe post-traumatic stress disorder (PTSD). This might include reactions such as diving under a table at a loud noise, being triggered to defensive or violent acts when startled, or languishing in depression. Traditional psychotherapy, which involves remembering the trauma, feeling the emotions, and passing through and beyond the trauma, did not work. In fact, these veterans became worse. Remembering the horrors of war reopened their emotional wounds, causing them to relive the traumas over and over again.

Why was psychotherapy so unhelpful? The part of the brain known as the *amygdala* shuts down during severe trauma. The amygdala is the bridge from the emotions to the cognitive centers. When it is blocked, the emotions alone drive behavior. No amount of mental effort can stop this reaction, because the emotions and thoughts have been disconnected. This automatic reaction is needed for survival when the bombs are falling, but an incapacitated amygdala continues to block the brain from dealing with events when the danger is past. Severe trauma leaves the brain in a state of shock. A generation of therapists, led by Francine Shapiro, developed forms of therapy that use eye movement or patterns of touch. One of these approaches became widely known in the mid-1990s as *Rapid Eye Movement Therapy*. This complementary therapy produces results. Brain scans performed before and after such therapies show that the amygdala is able to return to its natural functioning, so that a backfiring car becomes only a car making a noise, not a sound that triggers battlefield behavior. Energy healers can work as a team with psychotherapists trained in Rapid Eye Movement Therapy in order to help unblock the traumatized brain. Recovery comes much faster when the psychological and energy components are addressed.

Most psychotherapists and healers obtain information about emotional blockages by talking with their clients and listening to their stories. Images and memories of past events can be unblocked with the help of a neutral therapist: someone who can create a safe place of acceptance and who has no fear of being a companion on the journey and no attachment to the outcome of therapy. Once an atmosphere of trust and safety has been established, emotional blockages become so tangible they can almost be touched. Visions of a traumatic event may arise spontaneously from within. Detailed information can be useful in identifying the specific parts of the event that are most troubling so they can be addressed.

Peeling away emotional blockages allows
the true power of the self to emerge.

Gentle removal of the obstruction continues to deepen the clearing, allowing the brain to remake its normal connections. Peeling away emotional blockages allows the true power of the self to emerge. Gifts that were buried under the weight of these obstructions are free to be expressed and bring joy. What emotions block you? What ideas about yourself are no longer useful? What attitudes or beliefs do you hold that make you feel you are not worthy of receiving goodness in your life?

BRIDGE TO HEALING

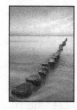 Reflect on the emotions or mental beliefs that are no longer useful to you. Perhaps at one time you found a certain belief or response necessary, but now it limits the fullness of your life or your expression of who you have grown to be.

Many naturally empathic people enter the healing professions with the highest humanitarian goals. After a while, the nurse becomes crabby, the doctor brusque, and the therapist jaded. Parents and caregivers seem susceptible to developing similar attitudes. Exhausted by the stress of absorbing the emotions of others and carrying them around day after day, we are at risk of experiencing total burnout. Meditations to clear blockages can rekindle zest for life and work. These benefits can be enhanced with healthful eating, exercise, and taking vacations.

BRIDGE TO HEALING

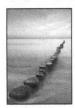

1. If you are prone to absorbing the emotions of others, make a list in your journal of the feelings you experience that are not your own—for example, undeserved anger toward the grocery clerk when the real problem is that your teenage son or daughter started an argument about telephone restrictions.

2. Use the images of the clouds covering Mount Baker on pages 66 and 67 as a metaphor for blocked feelings, either your own or those you have empathically absorbed from others. Allow your emotional blockages to float into the sky for transformation, as if you are removing the clouds from the mountain. Continue with a focused process of releasing each of the feelings you listed in your journal.

Clearing Physical Blockages

Elli hobbled into my office on crutches. She had made an appointment intending to work on other issues, but a recent skiing accident resulting in a broken leg occupied the focus of her visit.

Cell-Level Healing

It was the first time she had been to my office, and after going over her personal history, I helped her onto my treatment table. I use a massage table with a thick foam pad covered by a handmade quilt. Comfortable and relaxed, fully clothed, and covered with a soft blanket, Elli sighed with relief.

The first step in a healing session always involves searching for blockages. I held my hands about six inches above her body and moved them slowly from her head down along her arms, over her torso, and finally down each leg. My hands stopped at one specific place above the cast on her right leg as if a wall had leapt up. I asked Elli if this was the site of the break, and she said it was.

I attempted to clear the blockage, assuming the "stuck" energy was the result of trauma, but I could not seem to move past the area. As I continued to work on the blockage, an unusual sensation came over me. I could see the bones in Elli's lower leg. The two ends of the tibia were offset at the site of the break, as though her leg had not been set properly before casting. Imagine how odd I felt telling Elli that I had seen the inside of her leg and that she needed to seek further medical attention!

Two weeks later, we met again after an X-ray confirmed that her leg was misaligned. Surgery and titanium pins were needed to correct the position of the tibia. Later, as I cleared the energy from the surgery, I could feel energy flowing smoothly along her body. I focused on enhancing her natural healing process, and Elli recovered fully and returned to her active, athletic life.

• • •

Jeremy's injury was a different story. He had broken his ankle during a soccer game with his friends, all in their twenties. The ankle had healed as much as could be expected, according to the doctor, but he was still limping from pain eight months after the fateful game. Jeremy hoped energy healing would bring relief. After all, he was a young adult with many decades of life ahead, and he needed the full use of his ankle.

The orthopedic specialist had identified bone spurs as the culprits. He had done everything at his disposal: surgery for the original injury and months of immobilization in a cast. At this point, the doctor was out of treatment options and could offer Jeremy only pain medication.

Jeremy relaxed on the treatment table, his sock off and pant leg rolled up mid-calf. I began moving my hands above his injured ankle. After just a few minutes, his lower leg began to sweat and turned ghostly white. The rest of his body was normal. I felt spikes of sharp heat in my hands. As I continued to slowly run my hands above his lower leg, the spikes decreased and eventually subsided. We continued to work together in this way for several sessions until Jeremy's bone spurs were completely gone.

Osteoclasts are cells that remodel bone. They also have the ability to remove bone spurs. In addition to the healing work we did together in my office, I taught Jeremy to call his osteoclasts into action during meditation in order to achieve healing at the cellular level. In my development as an energy healer, I have learned how to reach into the body energetically to promote healing at the cellular level. I call this work *Cell-Level Healing*.

As a result of these techniques, his healing went far beyond what the physician had been able to do, and Jeremy returned to a fully mobile life that once again included soccer.

• • •

Physical blockages can occur anywhere in the body as a result of injury, infection, or disease. Removing the energy blockages does not necessarily cure the malady. However, it is a valuable first step to any subsequent treatment, because an open system with freely moving energy offers us the best chance of healing.

A range of sensations may indicate physical blockages in the body's energy flow. You may feel pain, heat, cold, or prickles. There may be no pain but rather an uneasy feeling that something is amiss. Blockages can be identified by any of the senses. Visual and auditory information might come in a vision, such as dense, red smoke, or as an anguished cry during meditation or the dream state.

Some of us inadvertently pick up blockages secondhand; we absorb pain from others and subsequently become ill. Releasing anything that is not your own increases your vitality and affirms the ability to distinguish between issues that are yours and those you have taken in from someone else.

BRIDGE TO HEALING

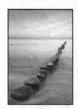

This exercise can be used to clear blockages and get rid of unwanted energy. Move your hands above the distressed part of your body while you visualize sending the unwanted energy into the earth for transformation or neutralization. You might also wash your hands in pleasantly warm water, mindfully washing away that which is no longer useful.

Clearing Blockages

Ancient practices that have been handed down for generations from other cultures can be useful when adapted to modern settings. One of these ritual ceremonies is particularly effective with physical blockage. In some shamanic cultures, even today, the healer or *shaman*—as did his great-grandfather before him—bends close to a subject's body and makes a sucking action with his mouth, either above the body or actually touching the body. In this way, he removes illness by drawing it out of the subject and into his mouth. The shaman immediately spits the spirit of illness into a small vessel, which is then smashed or thrown into a fire. This ritual unblocks the patient and calls forth the natural power of healing. The intent of the shaman is always to send the illness to a higher power for transformation.

BRIDGE TO HEALING

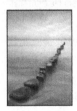

The shamanic healing described above can be adapted in several ways that do not necessitate an actual slurping sound. Here are two methods:

1. As demonstrated on page 68 in Your Bridge from Soul to Cell, simply visualize any blockage to robust health softening and flowing away like the natural phenomenon of ice melting in the winter sun.

2. Visualize filling the small ceramic or clay vessel on page 69 with the spirit or consciousness of illness. Gently gather the unwanted energy of these blockages. Ask for transformation of the

malady and removal of all negative impact. Find a ceremonial vessel and create a sacred place to clear yourself daily.

Clearing Spiritual Blockages

How do you know if you have a spiritual blockage? This is truly a complex question, because spiritual malaise weaves seamlessly into the emotional and physical areas of life. Release of a spiritual issue, when it is the primary blockage, may clear all the other levels, and then what we recognize as a miraculous cure takes place. I have seen this time and again. Not all ills are spiritually based, however, and attempting to cure everything from hangnails to cancer through spiritual clearing is not realistic. On the other hand, resolving spiritual issues can significantly support recovery from surgery, disease, and emotional trauma.

The signs of spiritual health include an inner peace so deep that none of the challenges of daily life can shatter the core tranquillity. Spiritually clear individuals awaken with joyful anticipation of each day. Meditation or prayer is as important to them as breathing and food. They easily shift from meditative stillness to the experience of oneness and ecstasy. People who are spiritually clear discover that they can live fully present in ordinary life while simultaneously maintaining a connection with their spiritual center. To illustrate, let me share with you a personal story.

Several years ago, at a time in my life when I was content with my healing practice, waking each day full of joyful feelings and enjoying the respect of my community, a yellow-jacket incident shattered my complacency. I was puttering around the yard at my

Clearing Blockages

Mount Baker cabin when three agitated yellow jackets stung me: two in the inside elbow area of each arm and one on the back of my neck. Large red welts swelled two inches across. They remained itchy and hot for weeks. Eventually requiring treatment with cortisone, an unstoppable rash crept from my arms to my shoulders, chest, and neck. Restful sleep was a distant memory.

Despite the cortisone treatments, the stubborn rash and discomfort persisted. Had the rash resolved fully with cortisone, there would have been no impetus to look deeper. In my distress, however, I chose to turn to the spiritual dimension to find meaning in this painful episode.

Healing means holding the lamp long enough to see God in everyone, to recognize the Divine in everything.

Knowing better than to ascribe a personal cause and effect to the yellow-jacket stings, I focused beyond the rash to the desired outcome, which was clear skin that did not itch. This focusing exercise evolved into a passage, a bridge with no return from my life afterwards to my life before. My energy shifted. My commitment deepened; my resolve to grow out of complacency strengthened. Not immediately, but soon, the rash receded, deep sleep returned, joyful waking moments returned, and I barely remembered the hot, red itching.

The spiritual healing I experienced came from within as I chose to see the episode as an initiation into new service. In addition, energy clearing from colleagues supported the transition back to health. Healing means holding the lamp long enough to see God in everyone, to recognize the Divine in everything.

BRIDGE TO HEALING

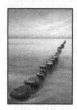 To help heal yourself spiritually and ease your way through any difficult passage, try this two-part exercise—yellow jackets are not required! Always remember that a world of flowing energy and blessing awaits you.

- Allow a deep connection to spiritual reality. There are many ways to find your connection: a moment of silence, a prayer, a special visualization. Perhaps an angel, a four-footed animal, a bird, or a spirit guide beckons you to start the journey. Pages 70 and 71 show two examples.

- Create a personal prayer or use the Jabez prayer, which follows, to affirm your willingness to grow. Say it repeatedly.

Practical Application of the Jabez Prayer

Lord, bless me, indeed. Before the day begins, before visioning and action, make a conscious choice to become still. Stay with this first line of the Jabez Prayer until your mind settles, becoming naturally quiet. Maintain your clear state by receiving this blessing at the beginning of each day.

Expand my territory. The connection to Spirit creates a natural flow of energy that is available for service. It shines with the true gifts of the individual. Expanded opportunities for service will show up unexpectedly as you pray the powerful second line of the prayer. The words "I'm willing" may be added.

Place your hand upon me. How many times have you embarked on a worthy project only to run out of enthusiasm before it's finished? Pray for sustained connection and energy in addition to inspiration. "Place your hand upon me" can sustain you and keep you on track.

Keep me from evil that I may do no harm. This line of the Jabez Prayer can be individually interpreted; for example, "Let me not waver from integrity in myself, my thoughts, and my actions."

Although different in interpretation, I thank Bruce Wilkinson for writing about the Prayer of Jabez and inspiring many people to look at I Chronicles 4:9–10 in a new way.

4

Flow and Soul-Signatures

**Ancient philosophies
call the energy of life by many
different names—among them *Chi.***
The robust flow of Chi is associated with vibrant health, whereas the absence of flow is correlated with ill health. A natural return to the unobstructed flow of Chi occurs when blockages are removed, allowing the body, mind, and spirit to be open and clear.

What is the nature of this flowing life energy? In my early work with clients, I could sense flow patterns—and, curiously, each person's felt different. The patterns were unique, much like fingerprints or snowflakes. In fact, I was able to recognize an individual and recall the issues we had previously addressed simply by noticing the particular signature of their energy flow.

*Each person embodies a distinctive variation
on universal energy.*

How could Chi be so variable? I wondered whether there was an "energy signature" that was a part of personal identity. Eventually, two principles emerged:

1. Each person embodies a distinctive variation on
   universal energy: a natural and unique pattern

exists for each individual consciousness. I call this quality their *Soul-Signature*.

2. In a healthy individual there is an abundant flow of energy through the body. In this regard I will use the word *Flow* to convey the quantitative aspects of speed and direction of the *Soul-Signature*.

Let's look at what Flow means to the cells from the point of view of the following fundamental fact about biological life: all cells experience a constant in-and-out flow of the elements necessary for survival. This essential pattern includes growth, repair, replication, response to stimuli, acquiring nutrients, and expelling waste. Scientists call this biological flow *homeostasis*, which literally means "a relatively stable state of equilibrium." This profound state of balance prevents sudden changes that could kill these delicate units of life. Complex feedback loops keep the cells at the correct temperature, regulate size, and maintain a relatively consistent molecular organization. Food and oxygen move into the cells, and waste is removed. Life ceases for a cell or group of cells without this Flow. If disease prevents large areas of Flow in a critical organ, the entire body dies.

The topic of Flow places us on that delicate threshold between spiritual, emotional, and physical issues. Well-established Flow changes a person's inner perception from empty to full, from waking in a state of dread to waking with contentment, anticipating the day ahead. Joy at simply being alive may prompt spontaneous outbursts of gratitude. When Flow reaches all of the levels from Soul to Cell, liveliness enhances simple daily routines. The body responds with improved health. Spiritual healing, therefore, works best in concert with the natural order of life.

Ed called me for an appointment because he was intrigued by the ideas I expressed about energy healing during an interview on Art Bell's *Coast to Coast* radio show. Ed had felt the chill of death when he nearly died during hospitalization for alcoholism. Fortunately, he recovered completely and no longer uses alcohol, but he was now faced with serious heart problems. Our first session seemed to have little effect. Intense concentration was required to clear enough of the stuck energy in Ed's body to allow him to feel any Flow. Fortunately, we both saw enough progress, albeit temporary, to continue. After a few sessions, Ed began to respond physically. His stamina increased and his fatigue receded. "I just feel better!" was how he described it.

We continued with individual sessions, and Ed also attended my classes to develop his own healing gifts. He enjoyed focusing healing energy on others and was quite effective in clearing blockages and increasing Flow in his fellow students. The results in his own body were significant; his health steadily improved. Ed's purpose in life was now expanded, and he volunteered each weekend at a local spiritual bookstore doing energy healings.

Our sessions continued on a monthly basis, with emphasis on supporting the Flow in his body. As his physical health continued to improve, he began to have extraordinary spiritual experiences. Sensations of floating, expansion, and great lightness came over him. He experienced joy and awe. Each session opened him to new levels, which were reflected in a profound evolution in his view of himself.

Our goal was to find a specific quality of energy and a Flow pattern that would stabilize Ed so that he would not become re-blocked after our sessions when confronted with the stresses of work and the ordinary trials of traffic, groceries, and his checkbook.

As I listened to him, I began to experience the unique energy that resonated within the very core of his being. Many experiences in my own journey had taught me to tune in to the particular energy imprint of the client. Ed had his own angels, his own guides, and his own healer's heart, but they were buried under years of creating himself as an astute manager and business person and an alcoholic. While working with Ed, I discovered something I have come to think of as each person's specific *Soul-Signature*.

Ed's way of seeing himself as an administrator did not support health in his body or peace in his soul. Ed felt wonderful when we uncovered his core energy. The next step was to stabilize the energy and to then teach him how to access his own Soul-Signature. Once again, I was reminded that energy work is most effective when it respects and harmonizes with the specific energy of the individual.

The Soul-Signature draws from three aspects of Flow that I will explain next:

1. An exact vibrational frequency that can be found as we peel away the beliefs and other blockages to our true self

2. The speed of Flow

3. The direction of Flow

The Vibrational Frequency of Flow

Our perception of color relates to the vibrational rate, or frequency, of the electromagnetic radiation received by our eyes. The entire universe is constantly moving at different rates of vibration. Not all of them produce color, because not all vibrations are within the rather narrow band of visible electromagnetic radiation. As biological systems, we are highly sensitive to light and color. This quality extends to our spiritual sensitivities. Indeed, color has been associated with healing for decades in esoteric teaching and for centuries in many indigenous cultures.

Color is often ascribed to the energy centers in the body (*chakras*) and to the energy field that surrounds the body (the *aura*). People who are able to perceive these colors are seeing with their *inner vision*: an altered state that allows a person to perceive images and hues not ordinarily seen by the physical eyes.

The Core Color is perceived as a cylinder of
light lying above the full length of the spine.

When I started working with color many years ago, I perceived deeper and deeper aspects of the body. I began to recognize the *Core Color*. The Core Color is perceived as a cylinder of light lying above the full length of the spine. As part of the Soul-Signature, the Core Color is more stable than the aura, not changing appreciably with mood or life situation. Is the Core Color a reflection of our true self, our very soul? I cannot fully answer that question, but I experience these beautiful colors as part of the uniqueness and the mystery of the self and the connection with all that is. Does this color change during our growth and development? I cannot answer that definitively either, but my observation is that nothing is static in our bodies or our souls and that we dance between the comfort of stability and the exhilaration of change as we grow. Vibrant and mysterious, the harmonic oscillations (frequency changes) of the universe reside within us. Our Core Color, a beacon of inner light, can be one of the sources of healing for our cells, translating the frequency vibrations of health to the body.

Table 1 illustrates some Core Colors and possible corresponding qualities as I experience them. I do not suggest that these are all

Table 1

Color	Attributes
White	Protected by divine intervention
Yellow	Strong mental ability
Gold	Compassion
Red	Vitality
Green	Physical health
Blue	Clarity
Indigo	Insight
Rainbow	Integration of earthly values and spiritual connection
Purple with flecks of silver or gold sparkles	Oneness

the colors or that the interpretations are perfect. I hope they inspire you to discover the concept of Core Color for yourself.

You may want to construct your own chart and notice your personal relationship to color.

BRIDGE TO HEALING

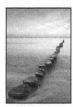

Here are some methods to use in identifying your Core Color:

- During meditation, you may see a bright color inside your head. Deepen your meditation to focus on the inside of your body in the area just above the spine. If the color persists, you can work with it as your Core Color.

- At times, you may be flooded with compassion, clarity, or insight, or all of these qualities at once. If there is an accompanying color, the quality and the color will be linked vibrationally.

- Someone else may become aware of your Core Color. This could happen during a session with a healer, for example. When you are in touch with your true Core Color, you will feel joyful, peaceful, and full of energy.

The Speed of Flow

The second quality of Flow is speed. Moving too quickly may feel jittery; too slowly will seem like nothing is happening. To be integrated, healing energy must move at close to the same rate as the client's Flow.

Imagine a small merry-go-round at a children's playground. You are going to jump aboard, but first you must run alongside the merry-go-round until you match its speed. Then you can grab onto one of the bars with your hand and jump up at the same time. Well executed, you will be sailing around with the kids. Miscalculation may leave you sprawled on the ground. In the same way, matching the speed of Flow will put you in perfect synchrony with compatible life-giving energy.

> *Matching the speed of Flow will put you in perfect synchrony with compatible life-giving energy.*

Use the following exercise to determine your optimum Flow speed. Please be aware that this may change from day to day, but you can always return to the exercise to find the correct speed for a particular task or life situation.

BRIDGE TO HEALING

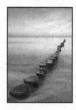

1. Flow speed varies with the time of day, life situations, and the basic nature of each person. Each time you meditate or stop to take a moment for yourself, notice how fast you are moving deep in your core. Note your personal Flow speed at that time.

2. When you are fully aware of your inner speed, notice whether it feels comfortable.

3. Conscious recognition of Flow will enable you to adjust the Flow speed to the optimum

level for each situation. Flow can be found where your fullest breath is found. Page 72, showing quiet water, and page 73, showing a rushing mountain stream, illustrate both slow and rapidly flowing energy. Where do you resonate?

The Direction of Flow

Many people read about Kundalini energy or hear a lecture on the subject by a spiritual teacher. Inspired by stories of amazing experiences of ecstasy resulting from the upward flow of energy from the base of the spine (*sacrum*), they try to "awaken" this energy in themselves and cause it to flow up their own spines. However, many people feel terrible with that direction of Flow—or frustrated that they cannot manage it once it happens. In twenty years of practice, I have found only a handful of people for whom an upward energy flow is healthy. Most of us flourish with Flow from the top down. This pattern could be called *spiritual homeostasis*, analogous to the flow of nutrients and energy that maintain life within your cells. What flows in also flows out, resulting in constant replenishment of energy and inspiration.

BRIDGE TO HEALING

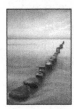
Visualize the crown of your head opening like a flower. Invite God's loving energy to flow into and through your body, supplying vitality to all of your cells. Then visualize the energy gently exiting through your feet.

How can you maintain the Flow you feel during meditation or after a session with an energy healer? Indeed, how can caregivers, parents, and empathic people maintain their own flowing energy? Jason's story serves as a good illustration as to how to maintain Flow.

Jason came to my office exhausted and discouraged with his work; but more than that, he was despondent about life. He was a professor at a university and thrilled to be a teacher and mentor, but he gave so much of himself to his students that he felt drained. His body hurt. Night after night, his painful knees, shoulders, and neck interrupted his sleep.

During his third session—after extensive clearing—he had a most unusual sensation. Energy was rushing through his body like water over a waterfall. The energy was so physical and strong that it tickled the soles of his feet. The pain left his body and his spirits lifted. He felt joyous and strong. We continued to work together for five weeks, and then we took a break. Many of the good effects were still present when I saw Jason again three weeks later, but a sense of discouragement and tiredness had begun to creep back. We explored the cause of his recurring negative feelings and found that a general climate of oppressive authority in his work environment was slowly shutting down his energy flow.

The process to reestablish Jason's inner sense of peace included the simple act of remembering the tickling sensation of the Flow, which had been so helpful before. Jason's practice of meditation, gratitude, and prayer, and a healthy lifestyle that included eating good food, exercising, and having a supportive community outside of work, further enabled him to avoid destructive energies.

Flow and Soul-Signatures

Cell-Level Healing enabled Jason to connect with the Flow of positive energy. Maintaining the Flow and building confidence to accomplish his own connections have been essential for his continued good health.

• • •

Connection with our personal
Soul-Signature always bestows healing.

There are hundreds of activities designed for protection that are supposed to prevent negative energy from disrupting the healthy or healing state, such as wearing amulets or saying magical words. I've probably tried them all! After a lot of disappointment, dashed hopes, and discouragement regarding techniques, I found that the only true stability and protection is the connection with Nature, Source, God, the Universe—however you name it. So often we focus on the people or issues that depress us and expend our precious life energy flailing in the mire of negativity. No one can avoid difficulties, but moving past them and reuniting with Spirit renews our life-sustaining Flow. Connection with our personal Soul-Signature always bestows healing.

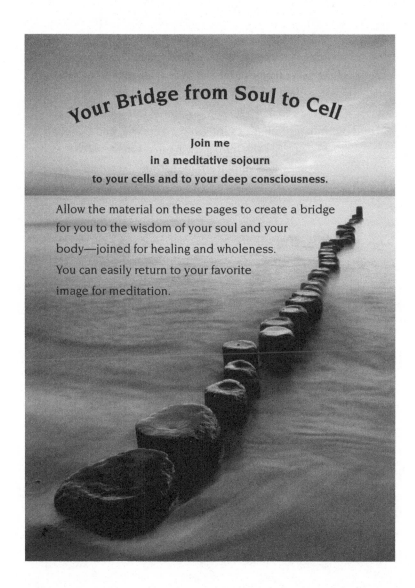

Your Bridge from Soul to Cell

**Join me
in a meditative sojourn
to your cells and to your deep consciousness.**

Allow the material on these pages to create a bridge
for you to the wisdom of your soul and your
body—joined for healing and wholeness.
You can easily return to your favorite
image for meditation.

Living systems show fractal
patterns that appear to grow from within themselves
expressing the same themes over and over again at their outer edges.
Patterns large and small
lead us to consider the wonder of our bodies
and our inherent qualities for growth, renewal, and healing.
Consider the fern, growing in a forest,
its leaf pattern repeating
again and again.

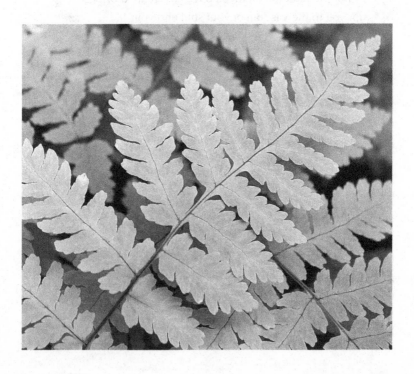

The salmon's gills branch
in a similar pattern as the fern.
This picture shows the microstructure of the
salmon's gills as seen through an electron microscope.

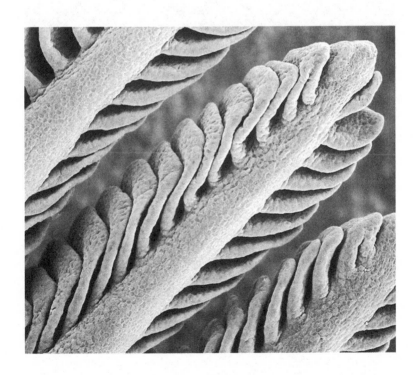

Cell-Level Understanding

Here is an electron micrograph of a sperm fertilizing an egg. We each begin as one sperm and one egg and develop into nearly 100 trillion cells. Personal bridges to healing stretch from our souls to our emotions and then through our minds to the teaming mass of our cells. On the next few pages you will become aquainted with cells.

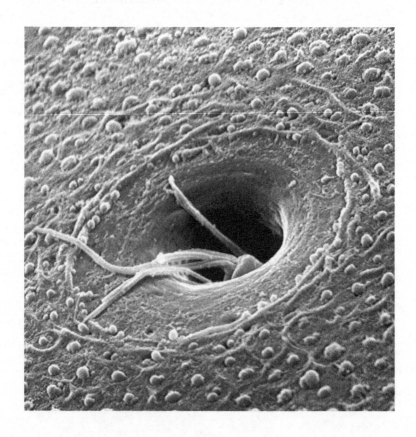

Cell Structure and Function

Cell structure and function are inseparable. Using the color code, you can identify cell parts that contribute to physical health.

Purple: cell membrane = communication
Green: endoplasmic reticulum = action
Pink: nucleus = DNA = information
Blue: mitochondria = power

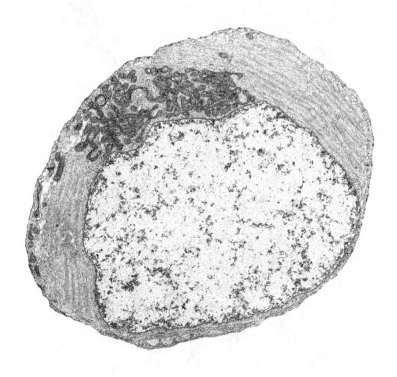

Comparisons of Healthy and Sick Cells

One cell nestled among its neighbors shows its internal structure. Notice how beautiful and organized the healthy cell below appears.

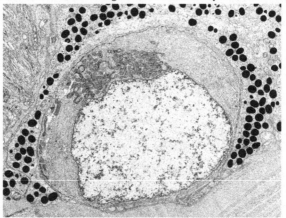

Sick cells lose organizational integrity as they lose function. The sick cell below is breaking apart into fragments that will be recycled.

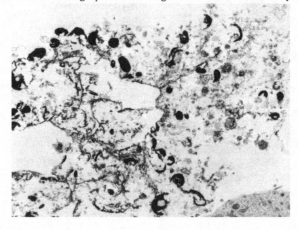

Healthy lens cells in the eye wrap around the circumference of the lens and allow light to pass clearly for good vision.

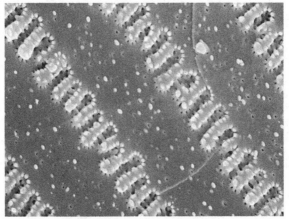

Lens cells in an eye with cataracts lose the beauty of their structure as sight becomes impaired or lost.

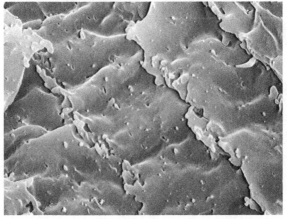

A family of cells called phagocytes, meaning "eating cells," clean up dead cell debris. One type of phagocyte—a macrophage—is known as "big-eater." Here a macrophage eats damaged connective tissue.

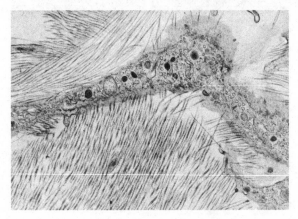

Macrophages create sacs containing material to be recycled, digest the material, and then make it available for healthy cells to reuse.

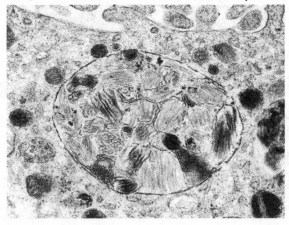

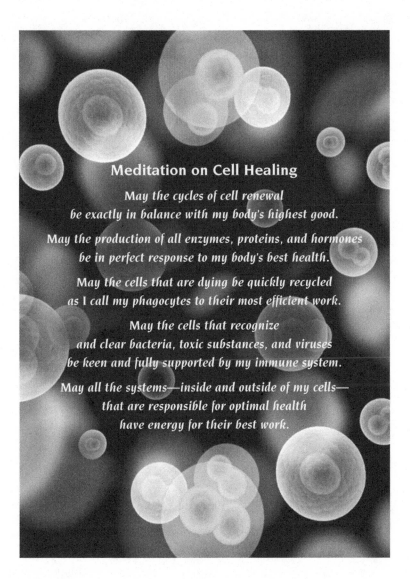

Meditation on Cell Healing

May the cycles of cell renewal
be exactly in balance with my body's highest good.

May the production of all enzymes, proteins, and hormones
be in perfect response to my body's best health.

May the cells that are dying be quickly recycled
as I call my phagocytes to their most efficient work.

May the cells that recognize
and clear bacteria, toxic substances, and viruses
be keen and fully supported by my immune system.

May all the systems—inside and outside of my cells—
that are responsible for optimal health
have energy for their best work.

Enjoy a healing interlude on the next six pages. You can use these images to clear your mind to become still and entirely present in the moment. Allow the words to gently filter through your mind, inform your spirit, and begin healing your cells.

Healing occurs in the manner of Creation:
Cell by cell
Shimmering
Coursing through the molecules
Stirring the waters to life

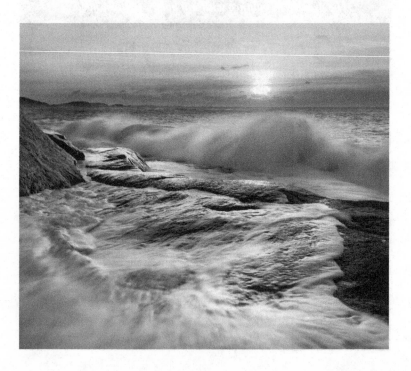

Breathe the breath of life into your cells as you imagine yourself opening to healing energy as a lotus opens to the sun.

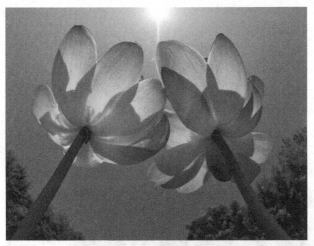

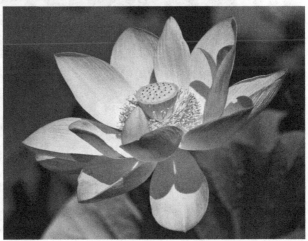

Practice of Appreciation

Observe a cell.
See the power of Creation.
See divine design.
See immense wisdom.
See the Heart of it All.

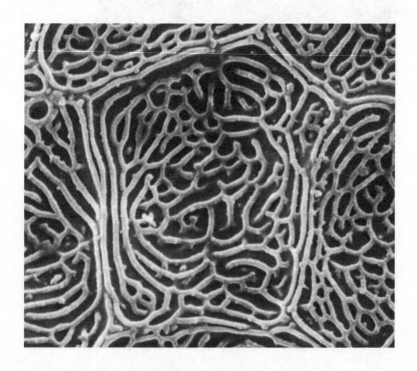

Look at a flower.
See divine design.

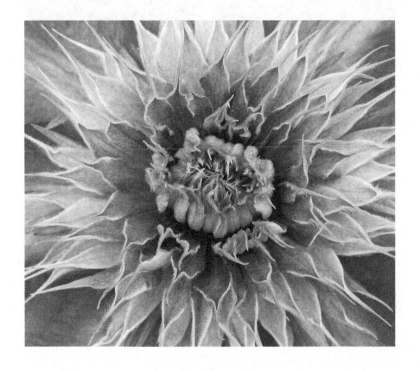

Behold a mountain.
See the power of Creation.

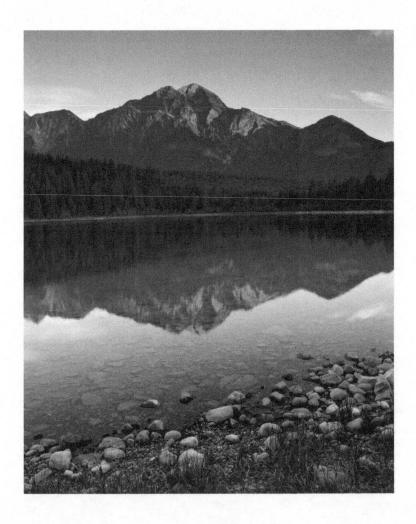

Consider a dragonfly.
See immense wisdom.

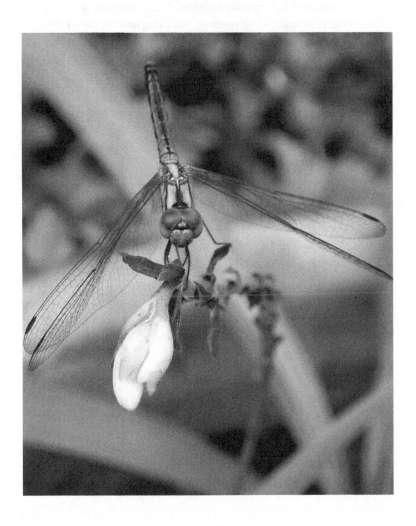

The universe is mysterious.

The universe is constantly creative.

The universe dynamically balances flow and organization.

The universe is resilient—constantly renewing and repeating itself.

As the universe, life is mysterious, creative, dynamically balanced, and resilient. Pause a while and enjoy the qualities of the universe of life. What universal qualities support your healing today?

Perhaps the mystery of a galaxy unexplored…

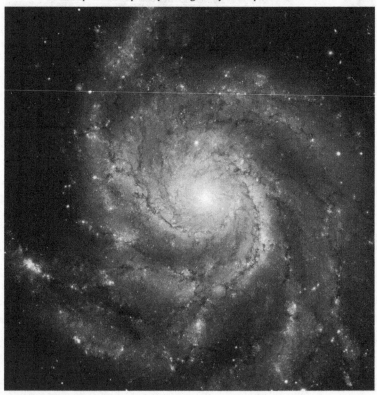

the creativity of seeds about to burst…

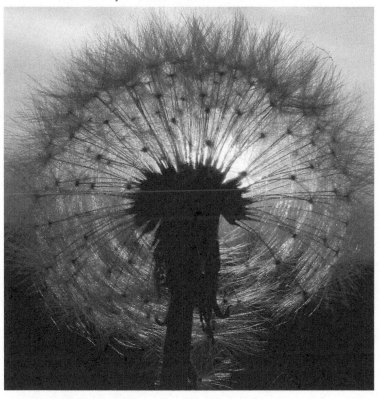

the dynamic balance of a changing landscape…

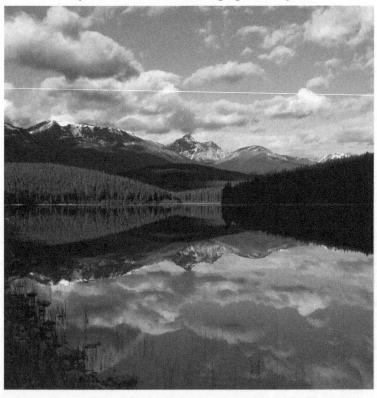

the resiliency of a flower blooming in the snow.

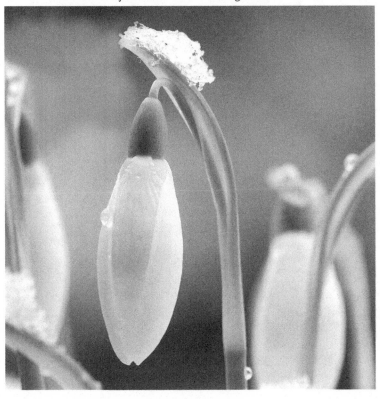

Releasing Emotional Blockages

In the following two pictures, use the first image of the clouds covering Mount Baker as a metaphor for blocked emotions—either your own or those empathically absorbed.

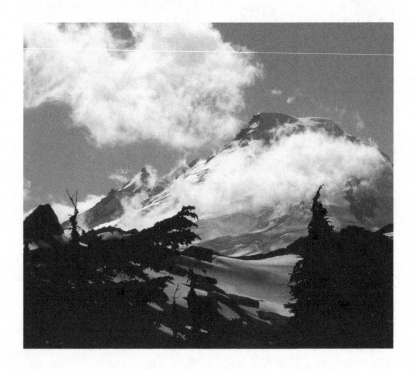

Allow your emotional blockages to float to the sky of transformation in the same way as the clouds float up from the mountain. Continue in a focused way releasing each emotion you would like to release.

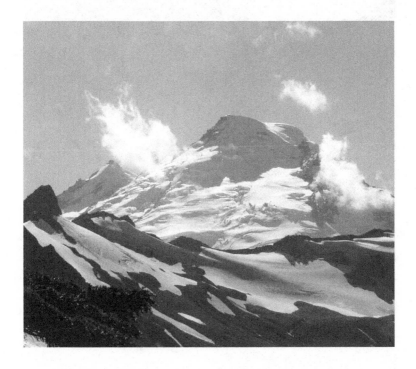

Clearing Physical Blockages

Two ways of clearing physical blockages follow. One involves working with the natural phenomenon of melting ice and the other with a sacred vessel.

Like ice melting in the winter sun, visualize any physical blockage to robust health softening and flowing away.

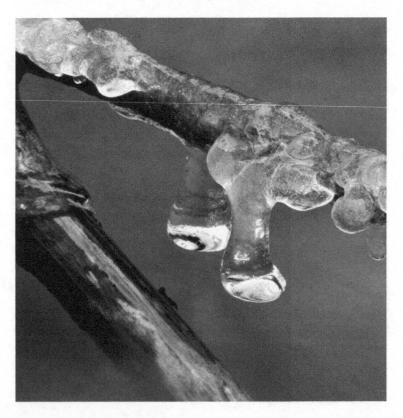

Visualize filling a vessel with the spirit or consciousness of illness or of any physically perceived blockage. Ask for transformation of the malady—represented by the white feathers—and removal of all negative impact. Find your own ceremonial vessel and create a sacred place in which to clear yourself daily.

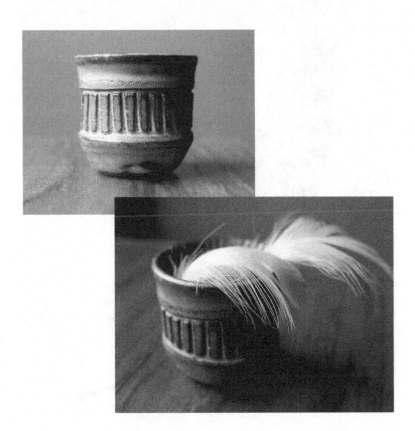

Releasing Spiritual Blockages

Allow a deep connection to your spiritual reality. Perhaps the image of an eagle will bring a sense of freedom to your spirit as you begin to lift above the heavy burdens of spiritual malaise.

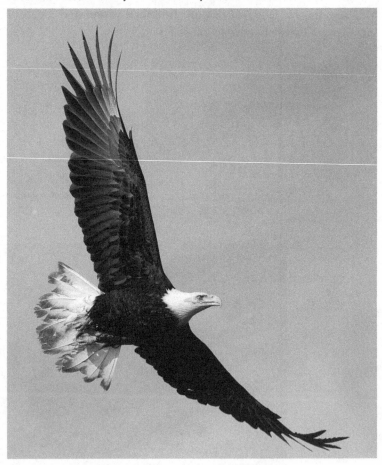

Allow your inner sense of Flow to stream from above your head downward as if you are standing under a warm, tropical waterfall.

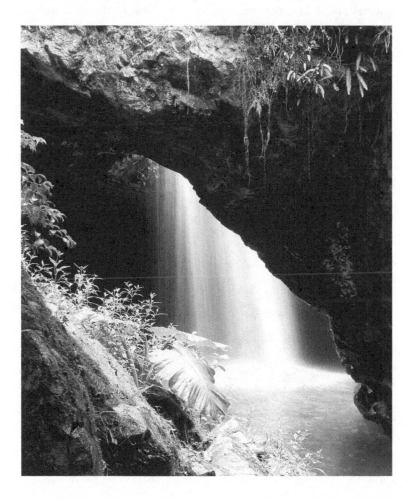

Finding Your Personal Flow Speed

Your rate of Flow will vary with the time of day, the situation, and your basic nature. Each time you meditate or stop for a moment for yourself, note your personal speed. Is it closer to the calm waters below, the rapids on the next page, or somewhere in between?

When you are fully aware of your Flow speed, think about whether it feels right for you. Consciously adjust this speed to what you need. If you were in a raft on the river below, would you choose to take the first quiet tributary or enjoy the rushing mountain stream?

Where do you resonate?

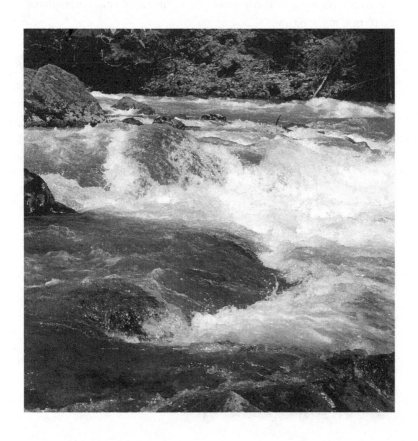

A Scientist Becomes a Healer

Cells are so small that 10,000 fit on the head of a pin, yet each cell does its part for the health of your body. In order to see into the world of minuscule cells, scientists use special microscopes that utilize electrons rather than light. The scanning electron microscope (SEM) images the outer surface of tissue samples. The transmission electron microscope (TEM) looks at the inside of cells, magnifying up to one million times.

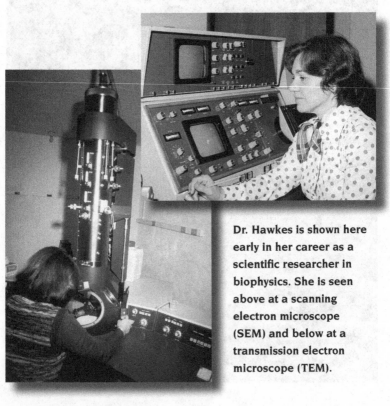

Dr. Hawkes is shown here early in her career as a scientific researcher in biophysics. She is seen above at a scanning electron microscope (SEM) and below at a transmission electron microscope (TEM).

A new consciousness brought on by a near-death experience in 1984 turned Dr. Hawkes's interest toward a life of healing. In the summer of 2005, Dr. Hawkes was invited to Dr. Akio Mori's state-of-the-art laboratory at Nihon University in Tokyo to have her brainwaves mapped by a 128-sensor electroencephalogram (EEG). Dr. Mori commented, "I have measured many people's brainwaves. Dr. Hawkes's brain shows a higher level of focus than I have ever seen before."

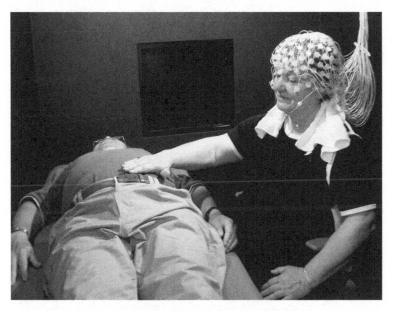

Electroencephalographic (EEG) testing of Dr. Hawkes's brainwaves during a healing session at Dr. Akio Mori's laboratory at Nihon University in Japan.

Quantitative electroencephalographic (QEEG) testing done by Juan Acosta-Urquidi, Ph.D., while Dr. Hawkes meditated and sent healing energy to a client three thousand miles away, showed how markedly the synchrony of her brain increased as many parts of the brain came together into phase during healing work.

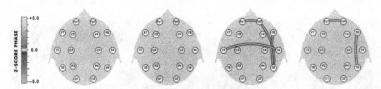

DELTA (0.5–3.5Hz) THETA (3.5–7Hz) ALPHA (7–13Hz) BETA (13–22Hz)

QEEG data plotted during ten minutes of baseline testing.

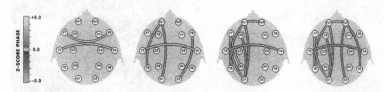

DELTA (0.5–3.5Hz) THETA (3.5–7Hz) ALPHA (7–13Hz) BETA (13–22Hz)

QEEG data plotted during fifteen minutes of remote-healing testing.

In 2006, Dr. Acosta-Urquidi again recorded Hawkes's brainwaves while working on two clients sitting about six feet in front of her. The data showed higher levels of focused delta waves, peaks of beta, and increased alpha during healing than seen in earlier testing. At the frontier of the science of neurology, the emerging field of neuroplasticity is providing insight for much-needed applications of the skillful use of our mind for cell-level healing. See the appendix.

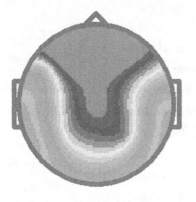

Quantitative electroencephalographic (QEEG) testing during a healing session with a client sitting in front of Dr. Hawkes. The bursts of delta brainwave activity more than doubled. The bright colors show intense brainwave activity.

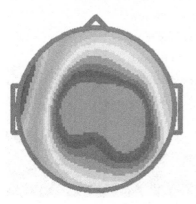

QEEG data show a dramatic increase in Dr. Hawkes's beta brainwave activity during a fifteen-minute healing session with a client. Alpha activity also increased (not shown here) on one side of the brain only.

Great Father, inspiration of Creation,

Great Mother, ocean of Emptiness,

Union of Joy,

Mystery beyond separation,

Having granted me

This precious Birth:

The burst of initial Light,

The body of your Oneness,

Grant me now, once again,

Your ineffable Oneness,

That I may be dissolved, yet

Reborn each instant,

Newly formed into Body,

Newly shaped by Light,

Instantly graced by Joy,

Naturally responding in Love.

Everywhere in time's

Dimension and discipline,

May we all find the Divine Interface...

Dissolving, as we began, into Bliss.

5

A New Look at Energy Centers

**It seems that in every class on healing,
after the briefest explanation of terms, the instructor
launches into a description of the seven classical "chakras."**
Some schools of thought include up to twelve. The colors, symbols, history, and methods for clearing these energy centers aligned along the spine suggest that everyone would be healthy, if only they could get their energy centers right. Years ago, I dutifully learned the system and then cleared, rebuilt, and made the energy centers glow with the proper assigned colors. Some of my clients felt superbly renewed, some felt nothing, and a significant number felt ill.

Energy Centers from an Alternative Viewpoint

The negative responses of some of my clients to the classical way of working with their energy centers prompted me to search for a new way to view them. Eventually, my practice changed, and I stopped imposing a certain vibrational frequency or color on any energy center. I watch, sense, and listen for the natural tone or color that is already present in the energy centers. If the tone is compromised by blockage, I clear the blockage and allow the inherent color to fill the newly opened space. This practice is another application of the Soul-Signature practice.

Cell-Level Healing

*Watch, sense, and listen for the natural
tone or color that is already present in the
energy centers.*

Some days my own energy centers are all singing in silver; other days, they are an array of different colors. If void of energy or muddy in color, I concentrate on the clearing phase of healing, followed by the Flow practices.

During the Flow phase, I enter the deep stillness of meditation, trusting the balancing energy of that state to take care of filling the cleared energy centers. I also ask for information and Divine guidance, if needed. A bright color may fill my mind, as a feeling of peace sweeps over me, or a shiver may float down my spine. These are all signals that the centers have been refilled. This alternative way of working with the energy centers has produced far better results than using the usual colors.

•　•　•

The healing journey of one particular client made me aware of the necessity to remain centered on what the client needs, *not* on how the energy centers are *supposed* to look. An aspiring Jungian analyst, Mike became ill with one viral infection after another. Barely able to function in his professional training program, and not helped by conventional medicine, he began exploring alternative approaches. Supplements made him sick to his stomach, or they had no effect. Acupuncture helped, but the benefits did not last. He sought my assistance as a last resort.

A New Look at Energy Centers

Our first session was discouraging. After Mike left the office, I meditated at length on his situation and prayed for guidance that would bring useful insights. My personal meditations are usually accompanied by vibrant purple hues that fill my mind's eye, but during my prayers for Mike, my inner perception sparkled with silver specks of light, like stars on a New England January night.

The issue was less about his energy centers and more about the color coursing up and down his spine. In my subtle (inner) vision, I saw a silver cylinder just above Mike's spine, stretching from his neck to his sacrum. This color was dynamic and sparkling. The ancient Hindu and Buddhist texts spoke of this cylinder, or channel, as the *sushumna*. In these texts, the energy centers were described as colorful wheels of light—each of these "chakra-wheels" were linked to the central cylinder and to the two parallel side channels called the *nadis*.

For Mike, our sessions using the color silver had a dramatic effect. He seemed to sigh with "silver relief" when I supported this color in his nadis and soshumna. His body easily overcame infection, and he was no longer sensitive to every whiff of environmental pollutant. As Mike learned to meditate while visualizing silver, his strength continued to improve. Once his condition was stable, we experimented with his visualizations by mixing a bit of red in his first energy center to support stamina, a touch of gold in the third for a strong sense of self, and some purple at his crown to enhance his meditations. Always keeping silver as the predominant color, he returned to health, professional stature, and a full life.

Energy Centers from the Classical Viewpoint

The standard energy-center locations, colors, and significances are usually depicted as shown in table 2.

Take a deep breath and allow your inner
focus to rest near your spine.

Table 2

Energy center	Location	Color	Significance
First	Base of the spine	Red	Holds vital energy for the physical body
Second	Belly button	Orange	Emotional body, relationships
Third	Solar plexus	Gold	How you are in the world, personal power
Fourth	Heart	Green	Compassion
Fifth	Throat	Blue	Expression, ability to communicate
Sixth	Between the eyes	Indigo	Insight and clairvoyance (inner vision)
Seventh	Top of the head	Purple	Connection to God

BRIDGE TO HEALING

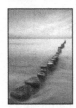

- Visualize filling your first energy center with red energy. Ask yourself: Does this color feel good? Does my body relax naturally with this chosen color? Is my spirit lifted when visualizing the color? If you have a positive response to these questions, proceed upwards to the next energy center and color and ask the same questions.

- If visualizing the classic colors described in table 2 does not accomplish something of value for you, try to determine your own Core Colors: Take a deep breath and allow your inner focus to rest near your spine. Can you intuit a particular color(s) that resonates with this deep core of yourself? If so, imagine sending the color(s) to each energy center, beginning with the first and working up to the seventh. Test your potential Core Color by asking the same questions as when you tested the classic colors (see above).

- People who are not visually oriented can work with frequency vibrations that are not restricted to the electromagnetic spectrum of light. For example, you may hear a sound or a tone resonating in your inner core, enabling you to sing your energy centers into alignment and balance.

- If the kinesthetic sense is easier for you, a tac-
  tile feeling of harmony in your energy centers
  may be the most accessible and powerful tool
  for balance.

As you continue to explore, trust that you will discover new aspects of yourself and new ways of finding balance and harmony as you respond to the challenges of daily life.

Simple Cell Basics

One of the basic tenets of biology,
one we all learned in school, is that all living creatures
are composed of tiny cells that can only be seen using a microscope.
We also learned that when one egg cell and one sperm unite they
start multiplying exponentially—two, four, eight—until they become
a sphere of cells that glows with the potential to form an entire body
with a liver, an eye, a big toe, or curly locks of auburn hair.

All living creatures are composed of tiny cells
that can only be seen using a microscope.

The cells of a salmon, a Labrador retriever, a statuesque elk,
and your own body look exactly alike. Indeed, all but one of the cell
photographs shown in this book are from fish, mostly salmon. Even
a trained electron microscopist cannot distinguish the inner structure of most kinds of cells from any species. Fish have some structures that adult humans do not have, such as gills, fins, scales, and
brightly colored dermal cells. Although these cells may appear different at one level of view, they display the same basic subcellular
parts that enable all cells to live. So when we talk about the inner
components of cells that generate power, action, information, and

communication, and we want a model that helps us envision our own cells, we can use these images of fish cells with confidence.

The cell-structure similarity between species is another facet of the oneness we share with all of nature, and the oneness within our-selves—the powerful mind-body-spirit connection that promotes health and healing. In a practical sense, the realization of the one-ness of all life can help us heal ourselves. Interestingly, we can also use the same energy consciousness to heal other species because their biology works in similar ways.

Over the years, I have had many cats and dogs brought to me by their owners. One dog was "Wolf," a gorgeous shepherd-wolf mix with a hole between two of the chambers of his heart, which could be heard as a severe heart murmur. Wolf's prognosis was dire; he would have to be put down. Elaine brought Wolf to me in her Volkswagen. He was not particularly sociable, and I had to go out to the car and slide into the backseat beside him. Wolf looked at me with great sus-picion as I began talking to him, reassuring him that I wanted to help him. He let me place my hand on his chest so I could send healing energy to his heart. After about eight minutes, he uttered a low growl. I knew the session was over.

Elaine returned with Wolf once a week for several weeks. He would wiggle a happy welcome, lick my face, and allow longer and longer healing sessions, always uttering that low growl when he had had enough. When Elaine took him to the vet after a month of treat-ment, the vet was astonished to hear Wolf's heart beating normally with no signs of damage. He lived a long and happy life with his owner. Wolf showed me how Cell-Level Healing can be used to help our canine friends and other companion animals.

Simple Cell Basics

From the smallest parts of our cells, a world of beauty and diversity has unfolded on this extraordinary planet, located on an arm of the Milky Way Galaxy at some wondrous longitude and latitude of the universe. We share this mysterious oneness at a deep level of structure, function, and consciousness. Although we cannot explain it, our recognition and experience of biological oneness can lead us beyond ourselves to embracing healing for our families, our communities, and our world.

Remote Healing at the Cellular Level

I could hear the strain in Teresa's voice on my voice mail. She spoke rapid, clipped English with a Canadian lilt and an exotic timbre. After several similar messages, we made a person-to-person connection, finally breaching the phone-tag loop. Teresa's mother, or *Muma*, lived in Jamaica. She could no longer walk to morning mass at the nearby parish. She was just too exhausted, but no one knew why. Life had stopped for Muma when this significant activity slipped beyond her grasp.

Teresa's older brother, Kwame, also lived in the Jamaican household. He suffered from diabetes and was experiencing the beginning stages of circulatory problems in his feet.

A time was arranged for me to call the family in Jamaica. After three rings, Kwame answered the phone. He spoke little English, and no one else seemed to be home. I could hear a rooster crowing in the background. Kwame and I exchanged greetings about a dozen times, until I simply said "Good-bye" and hung up the phone.

I decided the only way I could help Muma and Kwame was to go into a deep healing meditation and pray that it would link me to these charming people without the luxury of spoken language. This healing tool, *remote* or *distance* healing, is surprisingly powerful and effective at the cellular level.

Fatigue washed over me as I connected with Muma. I waited for guidance to let me know where to focus healing energy. Waves of fatigue plunged me deeper and deeper; ultimately, I felt like I was in the cells of Muma's body. If you could compare the energy contained in cells to light-bulb wattage, Muma was a 15-watt bulb, whereas a 100-watt bulb would be considered normal. Using the strongest Cell-Level Healing union I could manage, I linked to her and sent two pulses of energy. The first pulse turned her "wattage" up. The second began changing the information in her body to sustain the healing. Muma appeared clear, without much blockage, but she undoubtedly lacked Flow in her energy field.

> Remote *or* distance *healing is surprisingly*
> *powerful and effective at the cellular level.*

Kwame also complained of fatigue. However, unlike his mother, he had a confirmed diagnosis and was taking oral medication for diabetes. As I immersed myself further into the healing state, my focus was entirely on his pancreas. The cells responsible for insulin production seemed crippled. A powerful energy flowed through my body and across four thousand miles to Kwame—without the benefit of a telephone connection!

One week later, Teresa called to say that her mother had been able to walk to church two times the previous week and was hoping to get even stronger. Kwame's blood-sugar levels had stabilized, and he also felt more energetic and hopeful.

Simple Cell Basics

Over the course of the next six months, I sent remote Cell-Level Healing to Muma and Kwame once every five to six weeks. Muma continued to gain stamina, and she began walking to church every morning. I like to imagine her strolling with the soft morning sun on her back and the humid air infusing her every breath with the fragrance of sweet, tropical flowers.

Eventually, Kwame no longer needed medication for diabetes.

The Cell Is the Basic Unit of Life

Cells are the foundation of physical life. Groups of cells form tissues, and similar tissues join together and form organs, which are dependent on the health of the underlying cells.

Individually, cells are small: ten thousand can fit on the head of a pin. Yet if your cells were spread out like a galaxy of stars, they would occupy a space in the heavens a thousand times larger than the Orion Galaxy. Within each cell there are trillions of molecules composed of trillions more atoms. Like the spaces between stars, which contain huge amounts of energy, the ultrasmall nano-spaces inside of the atoms team with energy to constantly manifest new creation. In this microworld of the inner composition of your cells, energy and matter interface in ultrafast blips of time: nano- or picoseconds. When an event occurs in these swift pulses of 10^{-9} or 10^{-12} seconds, the cells enter a type of quantum reality—no longer linear and no longer predictable. The cell is the interface between ordinary and nonordinary reality; possibilities exist here that we have barely begun to understand or develop.

It's a good thing that we do not have to keep mental track of the operation of all these tiny parts. Yet we can influence them with our consciousness. Conventional research has established the detrimental effects of negative thinking, stress, and toxicity on the cells of the immune system and brain. Science has begun to offer evidence of positive thinking on the beneficial effects of spiritual practices such as meditation.[1] Improvements in health and happiness can be achieved by embracing the healing power of positive Flow.[2]

Hundreds of years ago, the poet Rumi put words to the mystery of the interconnectedness of soul and body when he wrote, "Soul, a moving river. Body, the riverbed." Cell-Level Healing happens at this interface of soul and body.

> *"Soul, a moving river. Body, the riverbed."*
> —Rumi

There are five components of cells that need to be understood in order activate your intrinsic capacity for renewal and healing. The scientific names of those parts unwittingly hide the amazing functions they provide. Each one has a crucial and defined function, as shown in table 3 and the photograph on page 51.

Most living cells share similar basic components and biological functions, although they may differ significantly in appearance. A single animal cell may be round, cubic, columnar, or long and stringy, depending on its location and particular job. Each cell has

1. Daniel Goleman, *Destructive Emotions: A Scientific Dialogue with the Dalai Lama* (New York: Bantam, 2004).

2. Goleman, *Healing Emotions: Conversations with the Dalai Lama on Mindfulness, Emotions, and Health* (Boston, Mass.: Shambhala, 2003); Gene Cohen, *The Mature Mind* (New York: Basic Books, 2005).

Table 3

Cell part	Structure	Function
Cell membrane	Complex cell boundary with receptor sites	**Communication:** Helps to regulate cell activity by allowing the passage of specific materials in and out of the cell and maintains structural integrity of the cells
Nanotubes	Ultrasmall extensions of the cell membrane that reach out to neighboring cells	**Communication:** Transfer information between cells via biochemical packets
Nucleus	Membrane-enclosed sphere inside the cell which contains DNA—the instruction manual for all of the body's needs	**Information:** Preserves the "codes of life" and regulates cell activities by producing templates for the manufacturing functions of cells
Endoplasmic reticulum	Long layers of specialized membranes in the interior of the cell	**Action:** Responsible for the final production of structural and enzymatic proteins
Mitochondria	Tiny powerhouses in cells surrounded by a double membrane with a small strand of its own DNA that contain enzymes for Kreb's cycle and ATPase	**Power:** Produce all the energy that cells need

an outer *membrane*, to which receptor molecules attach. These sites grab free-floating messenger molecules, such as hormones, and help push them inside the cell in order to trigger specific cell activities. This is one of several ways in which cells stay in communication with the rest of the body and adapt their biochemistry accordingly.

Plasticity, an attribute of animal-cell membranes, contributes to the soft nature of our bodies—compared to the crunchy cell walls of plants, which are fortified with cellulose. Trees could not remain standing if they had pliable animal-cell membranes. Only plant cells have walls that protect their cell membrane. In animals, the cell membrane can send tiny, fragile tubes to neighboring cells. These tubes are called, appropriately, *nanotubes*. Using this mode of communication, nanotubes send molecular messages to their neighbors, who, in turn, send nano-bridges to adjacent cells. Our bodies are vibrant, interconnected denizens of the universe, not 100 trillion cellular islands of isolation.

Inside the cell membrane an entire cosmos of complexity and beauty lives in the watery medium of the cell sap, the *cytoplasm*. More than 90 percent of the cytoplasm is water, and one can only speculate how our thoughts might affect this cell-water and thereby affect the critical life functions of the other subcellular components. Masaru Emoto's provocative work certainly challenges us to consider the messages we give our own watery milieu.[3] Floating fibers in the cytoplasm create a loose inner skeleton for stability, yet they allow Flow throughout.

3. Masaru Emoto, *The Hidden Messages in Water*, translated by David A. Thayne (New York, N.Y.: Atria Books/Beyond Words, 2005).

Simple Cell Basics

The *nucleus*, enclosed in its own membrane, occupies a good portion of each cell. Molecular pores punctuate the nuclear membrane for the passage of rather large arrays of molecules, which translate the directives of the genetic code, DNA (deoxyribonucleic acid), into cell production and function. DNA is the informational center of the cell.

Messages carried by molecules direct the assembly sites of the cell to make very specific substances needed by the body. These sites of assembly lie outside the nucleus in the *cytoplasm*. There, long sheets of folded membranes called the *endoplasmic reticulum* comprise the "action" part of the cell. Massive numbers of *ribosomes* spin from the surface of the endoplasmic reticulum. On these sites, molecular information from the nucleus directs the action of plugging one atom into another, thereby forming molecules in precise sequences, which then become proteins. Each protein is unique. One will become a muscle fiber; another, an estrogen molecule, an enzyme for digestion, or a protein that will partially shape your nose.

DNA is the informational center of the cell.

Cells may also export products into the bloodstream to be circulated to another part of the body for use. Neatly packaged in *vesicles*, these products are wrapped in their own membranes. They float to the cell surface and make their way out of the cell.

How does a cell obtain energy for all this work? After food is digested and absorbed into the bloodstream, cells take in what they need for the power stations of the cell to spring to life. Tiny ellipsoid dynamos, hundreds of the power-station-like *mitochondria* inhabit each and every cell. Magnificent, linked complexes of enzyme chains called the *Kreb's cycle* buzz in each mitochondrion, further breaking down glucose, one of the end products of food digestion (*glycolysis*), and releasing energy. As the bonds between carbon atoms in the backbone of glucose are unplugged, energy is released and then stored for future needs. This crucial energy does not run rampant, gleefully tripping through the cells, but rather it is instantaneously taken up by yet another type of enzyme (ATP*ase*), which hangs on the inside of the mitochondrial double membrane like a bat on a cave wall. Safely sequestered, the stored energy is available to the cell for heat, structural repair, or synthesis.

Curiously, the ATPase enzyme, which captures and releases energy, spins as it works. In fact, the universal spiral is resonant in every cell. The most impressive telescopes look outward and see spiral galaxies, and the most powerful electron microscopes look inside cells and see spiral structures smoothly running the business of life. The ribosomes perched on the endoplasmic reticulum arrange themselves in a spiral as they create all of the life-dependent proteins in the body.

DNA is packaged in a double spiral, and now we know that the enzyme responsible for all energy maintenance in the body spins as it works in the mitochondria.

Meditation Using the Universal Spiral Archetype and Cell Basics

The following meditations will assist you in visualizing the spirals of DNA and lead you deeper into the spiral archetype in order to connect you to the universal energy of Cell-Level Healing. Allow these universal spirals to support, renew, and energize your cells.

BRIDGE TO HEALING

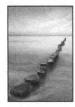

Imagine that you can reach a spiral galaxy and grasp a string of spinning stars.

Pull the twinkling spiral to your body. Anticipate that the cosmic spirals resonate with the spirals deep within your cells. Allow the universal spin to support, renew, and energize the components of your cells.

To go deeper, visualize the components of your cells and meditate on the following affirmations:

Cell membrane. May the boundaries of each of my cells be perfectly safe yet permeable, individually competent yet responsive to *communication* from my whole body.

Nanotubes. May *communication* from cell to cell be easy and accurate and may it connect throughout my body.

DNA. May all the *information* in my DNA be coded and translated for abundant health.

Endoplasmic reticulum. May all the enzymes and structures of my body resonate with health for optimal *action* in my body.

Mitochondria. May the spin of energy in my life emanate smoothly and plentifully—and with exactly the right amount of *power*.

7

Cell-Level Healing in Practice

**Whether our purpose is to maintain a state of
robust health or face an illness, our journey into the cells
opens the way for spiritual healing to influence our physical life.**

As our lives unfold, we experience challenges: injuries to body, emotion, and spirit. Some "scraped knees" remain scarred long past the expected healing time, and we need clearing of blockages to move beyond the limitations and mini-deaths they impose. Once clear, the flow of life-energy can fill us, sustain us, inspire us, and heal us. A new awareness of the deep reach of healing flow to the cells allows us to address our cells: the place where energy and matter interface to create life. At this interface, the dance of energy and matter equals the universal dance of unbounded spirit and the coalesced consciousness we call *physical reality*. Our cells and their exquisite inner workings choreograph and perform the dance.

*The cells are the place where energy and
matter interface to create life.*

The Guiding Principles of Cell-Level Healing

Before we discuss specific applications for Cell-Level Healing, let's examine the following guiding principles for healing:

Cell-Level Healing

1. *Pay attention*

   - Develop a profound level of appreciation for your body, mind, and spirit as well as gratitude for whatever state of life and health you now experience.

   - Identify blockages and proceed to clear them as best you can.

   - Use imagery and kinesthetic awareness to feel a flow of energy throughout your body to whatever extent is possible at any given moment.

2. *Notice resistance*

   - Notice if you are resisting anything in your journey to healing. This allows you an additional bit of time to focus on how clear you are and how available you are for healing.

   - If you find resistance, repeat the clearing phase until you sense flowing energy running into the crown of your head, down through your body, and out of your feet. Ask yourself for information about any resistance in a neutral, nonjudgmental way. This will allow you to either move on or to receive additional spiritual help to free yourself from any unwanted situations.

3. *Look within*

   - Turn inward and enter the safest and deepest state of meditation possible.

- The first part of your meditation should be simply finding a place of silence, followed by allowing intuitive wisdom about your situation to arise.

- As you turn inward, seek to identify the particular cells most in need of healing. Envelop those cells within an image of spirals made from soul-light. Hold this thought for as long as you feel fully engaged.

4. *Integrate healing energy*

- After completing a healing meditation, rest for a few minutes, holding the intention of allowing the healing energy to integrate throughout your body. Address the cells of your body, saying,

   "I trust you to continue healing, and I ask the spiritual dimension of my deepest healing consciousness to guide, sustain, and enliven you."

   Modify this statement in any way that works best for you.

We've looked at how living beings are ordered, yet remain fluid, and how the application of healing modalities must blend with the specific nature of our bodies. The application of spiritual healing as an adjunct to treatment for specific conditions requires paramount attention to individual situations and needs.

Following are a few examples of specific conditions in which Cell-Level Healing has been a positive influence. The accompanying meditations and visualizations have proven effective as an adjunct to medical and psychological treatment with hundreds of clients in my private practice.

This is not a comprehensive list of diseases or procedures that can be positively influenced by Cell-Level Healing, but rather it offers examples of how to integrate information about the body and the cells with healing meditations.

Aging

Is any process more natural and, at the same time, more fearfully loathed than aging? Witness the booming anti-aging industry, a cornucopia of cosmetics, supplements, and treatments designed more to calm our fears or fuel our fantasies than heal the damage from destructive factors such as unmitigated stress, sedentary lifestyles, and consuming an excess of fatty foods. What are the biological factors related to aging? How much influence do we have in achieving a long life and good quality of life?

As we discussed earlier, each differentiated or specific cell population has a rate of cell death and renewal that is genetically determined. Some cells of the body live a month, some stay with us our entire life span. Our human cells have the capability of renewal and repopulation when damage occurs.

Certain aquatic animals are made up of a limited number of cells, which form inside the egg case and completely cease dividing once the egg hatches. These simple creatures die when their limited number of cells wears out; their life is brief and predictable. They inhabit pond water and furiously swim about, whirring two rotors of cilia on their heads. Indeed, they are called *rotifers*, because of their unique way of locomotion. The biological principle illustrated here is that cells are programmed to live only a certain amount of time. Causes emanating from the codes of limited life, not predators or toxins from outside, bring the specter of death to the cells. *Apoptosis* is the biological term that refers to programmed cell death.

In humans, however, the situation is more complicated. We live much longer than rotifers, and we have many cellular systems with differing life spans. Rotifers are clear as crystal: we can see their cells through our microscopes. Our opaque skin makes it hard to see what is going on inside our body as we age. We know that our cells have a limited life span too. Red blood cells live for about 120 days and are continually replaced at the rate of three million a second. Molecules from cells that have worn out and disintegrated are garnered from the blood stream by the spleen to be recycled. Truly, we are an ultimate recycling project, using not only atoms and molecules from within but also from the beginning of time to create new cells.

If aging is such a natural process, then why include it in a discussion on healing? Two reasons emerge. The first is the uncertainty about how long humans can live under optimal conditions. Records indicate that some members of tribes living in the high Himalayas live reasonably well at 120 or more years. The second reason includes recent research on cellular damage that causes us to age earlier than our genetic programming. Given the journey we share with all life forms, a journey that eventually leads to death, the goal is to create optimal longevity and health on the journey.

For our own practice of cellular health, we look at the power pack of the cell: the mitochondria. These tiny ellipsoid energy centers contain their own DNA, albeit a small strand that has limited codes. When a cell divides to form two new cells (the process of renewal), the mitochondria also divide independent of the nucleus. They keep dividing and thereby repopulate the new cells with enough power centers to energize each cell. With aging, the short DNA strands in the mitochondria incur errors or mutations. Some of these significantly damage the integrity of the codes and eventually stop the production of new mitochondria. Cells die without energy to sustain them, resulting in tissues that either quit working or become highly impaired. For example, muscle mass declines with aging, most likely from such a mechanism. Cell death caused by mitochondrial damage appears to be more important in aging than stress, at least in mice, the animal used in this research.[1]

BRIDGE TO HEALING

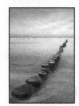

Here is a cell-level meditation for a healthy life:

1. Clear your mind of fear about aging. Envision a flow of energy throughout your body that is timeless, as it has been since the beginning of creation.

2. Embrace that energy with your body and consciousness in a relaxed manner. Envision it reaching into and simulating all of your cells.

---

1. G. C. Kujoth et al., "Mitochondrial DNA Mutations, Oxidative Stress, and Apoptosis in Mammalian Aging," *Science* 309 (2005): 481–84.

3. Visualize healing energy entering into the power centers of your cells and then even deeper into the small information strand of DNA in each mitochondria.

4. Ask that the information be secure from damage of any kind.

5. Send a boost of energy to your cells, with their precious codes for full function, full integrity, and full ability to renew themselves.

Arthritis

Arthritis results in inflammation that affects the joints of the body, including the fingers, wrists, knees, ankles, hips, and neck. There are two types of arthritis: *osteoarthritis*, a condition wherein calcium is deposited at the joints, enlarging and deforming the joints; and *rheumatoid arthritis*, an autoimmune condition wherein the joints often remain continually swollen and painful. The inflammation seems to travel from one part of the body to another, wreaking havoc wherever it lands. The cause of arthritis is not fully known, but injury, infection, or genetic predisposition is often indicated.

The specific types of cells involved in arthritis can be grouped into two categories: those that create calcium deposits and those that create the inflammatory response. The healing meditations for both types of arthritis include working with the two separate cellular events of bony deposition and/or inflammation. Inflammation causes pain, and without some relief most people with arthritis find it extraordinarily difficult to enjoy life.

BRIDGE TO HEALING

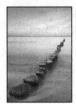

Here is an exercise for calcium deposits:

1. Osteoclasts can recognize the unnecessary calcium knobs, shards, and spicules that tear the soft tissue and exacerbate the inflammatory response. Call the osteoclasts in your body to an imaginary "board meeting" and announce that their top priority is to seek out unnecessary calcium deposits and completely remove them.

2. Trust that the genetic coding of the osteoclasts will restore to your body the optimal amount of bone and the proper distribution of calcium.

BRIDGE TO HEALING

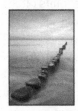

Here is an exercise for inflammation:

1. Imagine that your breath can reach the painful places in your body and linger there, softening the hard edge of pain so that you can subsequently release some of the pain as you breathe out. Repeat this until you feel you can move to the next step.

2. Imagine a cool mountain waterfall pouring through your body and washing over your hot joints, carrying the inflammation down and out through the bottoms of your feet. Visualize the

cells that respond to the inflammatory signals beginning to slow down and return to normal patterns of quiescence. Visualize them remaining quiet until they are truly needed to fight a specific illness.

Imagine a cool mountain waterfall pouring through your body and washing over your hot joints, carrying the inflammation down and out through the bottoms of your feet.

Autism

Autism has become a condition of increasing concern as more and more children are afflicted. The cause is unknown. The complex array of disability in autism usually shows up early, within the first three years of life. Current estimates indicate that one child in 250 is born with some form of the autistic spectrum. This neurological disorder results in impairment of language and speech, and it subsequently affects connection and communication with others. Although 70 percent of autistic children test below normal in intelligence, it is hard to know if this adequately reflects their cognitive function. Some of these children are dramatically bright and have highly specialized and focused intelligence.

In seeking any form of healing, parents and caregivers usually intervene on behalf of the child in the beginning, because of the young age of the child and the communication difficulties.

Cell-Level Healing

Two general issues have surfaced in my limited, but unusually successful, work with three autistic children. Two of them were five-year-old boys: one I met in person, and one, Terry, I did not meet. I had no direction connection with the third child, who was almost three years old and lived in the Midwest.

Terry's story started with his father calling me from Ohio to ask if I would try to help his son. I began to work with Terry in my meditation each morning to see if he would respond and whether I would be able to help him. At that time, two years ago, Terry was noncommunicative and almost entirely locked inside his own world, which included a fascination with automobiles.

For a period of two years, I conducted remote healing sessions with Terry. I would call his parents at the appointed time and then work with Terry remotely for about an hour. He is now talking, laughing, having birthday parties, and going to school. Although he is not entirely recovered, Terry has come a long way out of his withdrawn state. A highlight of one of our sessions was when Terry actually spoke with me on the phone.

When I meditated on all three children, at different times, I felt as if I was sequentially linked to their perceptions. When I was in that state of mind, I felt the children's confusion and distress. They felt overwhelmed with input, as if a hundred televisions were blaring at them all at once. It seemed that the noise and concomitant bewilderment frightened them and pushed them into whatever place of quiet they were able to find. I felt that "gates" were needed to control the level and variety of input. The first phase of my work was to create some safety for the child by "showing" them, using my own mind, the use of such safety gates.

Much later, when their parents reported that they were more relaxed, more communicative, and stable emotionally, I began to help them focus on one "channel" at a time. My hope was that they would learn how to limit the cacophony impinging on their consciousness. The final step was to invite them to explore the world beyond their gated isolation.

BRIDGE TO HEALING

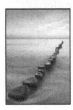

This exercise is for parents of children with autism. You will know best how often to work with your child. Initially, I suggest twice a week. In the beginning, you may see only subtle changes. Terry's first distinct step was a full-blown tantrum, but his parents were ecstatic. He had taken the lid off his tightly held emotions.

1. Without changing what your child is doing (including sleeping), and without invading the child's physical space, make a heart-level, spiritual connection between you and your child. Enter into a meditative state and picture your child, feeling the heart connection. You do not need to be physically near the child, because spiritual connections are not dependent on spatial proximity.

2. Imagine yourself in the safest possible scenario until you feel peaceful and safe yourself. Send thoughts of safety and companionship to your child, offering reassurance that the

child, too, can be safe in the world. Affirm that you will accompany and protect the child along the way and in every way possible.

3. In your visualization, show your child how you focus on one thing at a time, effectively blocking out a myriad of simultaneous inputs. Imagine approaching a television set and selecting only one television station, or looking at ten books and picking up only one. Send this image to your child using your mind, not words.

Cancer

Cancer cells are part of your body. At one time, they functioned perfectly well as a normal part of your breast, lung, pancreas, prostate, skin, or other tissue. Each cell has its own biological clock that controls its individual rate of repair, replication, and death. For example, skin cells live for about a month; red blood cells live for about four months; and nerve cells live for decades, if not your entire life. For mostly unknown causes, a cell of any tissue type may divide too fast and at random, resulting in a tumor.

A cell of any tissue type may divide too fast
and at random, resulting in a tumor.

An enzyme called $p53$ has the enormous job of regulating the timetable for cell division in normal cells. If a cell goes berserk and does not conform to the timetable, p53 first locks onto the DNA and re-regulates the cell. If that does not work, the cell will die. Cancer cells lack p53 enzymes. They also lose some of the distinguishing characteristics of their parent tissue; they de-differentiate and become strangely embryonic in structure. However, they retain enough of the qualities of the specific tissue to be recognized by a pathologist. When a tumor metastasizes to another location in the body, the original tumor location can usually be identified from the characteristics of the wandering cells.

Healing meditations for cancer derive from two types of information: (1) cancer cells are out of balance with the body and (2) cancer cells lack a crucial regulatory enzyme.

BRIDGE TO HEALING

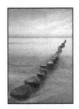

This exercise reaffirms cell balance:

1. Address the renegade parts of yourself, embracing them with your heart energy, emotions, and inner vision.

2. Send thoughts of conscious recognition and connection to the renegade cancer cells. Require that these cells either recycle (as in *die*) for the higher good of the whole body or return to the proper division rate for their tissue type. Tell all of your metastasized cells, "Recycle. Your molecules are needed for life to continue."

3. Accompany your in-breath with the thought "Balance" and your out-breath with "Harmony." Send this message for ten cycles to both your cancerous cells and your normal cells.

4. Genetic codes in the DNA of your cells retain the information to synthesize p53 for proper cell growth rates. Visualize a wave of energy moving from the top of your head throughout your body. Call forth the production of p53 once again in every cell. Enlist your p53 to work effectively and normally within its particular role for maintaining cell health in all tissues and organs.

5. Ask the nanotubes to network with all cells and transmit packets of information needed to synthesize their own p53.

Cancer is a complicated disease, and the method of using healing meditations for cell balance and the re-establishment of regulatory enzymes needs to be adapted to each individual's particular circumstances and personality. The following stories illustrate different ways of working with the basic principles described above.

Cindy was at the top of her game: a university professor, world traveler, and successful in everything she chose to do. To her dismay, she discovered a lump in her left breast. Had it grown so large overnight, or had she been too preoccupied with the overseas exchange program and her participating students to have lost track of her body? Tests confirmed there was a lump the size of an egg yoke high in the upper left quadrant of her left breast. A colleague who knew of my work encouraged Cindy to make an appointment with me before her biopsy date.

Cell-Level Healing in Practice

We had time for only one session before her biopsy. During that session we talked about bringing her body back into balance and harmony. We asked the cancer cells to recycle by dissolving and to consolidate in one place where it would be easy for the surgeon to remove them. The biopsy day arrived, and Cindy was well prepared and actually relaxed. She handled the procedure easily using her new tools of calming meditation and visualization.

The surgeon was quite surprised when she checked the original ultrasound. The tumor was now the size of a pea, much smaller than measured previously. The margins were clean and there was no indication of any involvement beyond the pea-sized tissue she had removed during the biopsy. The only conclusion the surgeon could draw was that the original ultrasound was inaccurate. Cindy, her family, and I celebrated her excellent prognosis, and we left the surprise and confusion about original tumor size at the doctor's office along with her medical chart. What mattered was her health—not trying to prove that spiritual healing shrinks egg-yolk-size masses to pea-size.

• • •

Anna called me in desperation. She had returned home from the hospital and was bedridden, in pain, and totally exhausted, whereas normally she was dynamic and endlessly energetic. Ovarian cancer had struck her suddenly, and it was found to be only partially operable. She had an astonishingly aggressive tumor that had spread all over her intestinal area, attaching to the omentum (a large membrane covering the intestines). Metastases had begun to grow in her liver and spleen.

Cell-Level Healing

She was not strong enough to come to my office, so I arranged a time for a house call. Lying on the couch, pale but determined to survive the cancer, Anna was ready to accept any information or help I could provide. Our first session included suggestions for breathing into the pain, softening it, and breathing it out. I also encouraged her to take pain medication so she could sleep and allow her body to recover from the surgery. Strong people who work in health-related professions are often the most difficult patients!

Relaxation imagery helped Anna over the next week, until we met again. By then, she wanted information on how to practice healing meditations. We talked about balance and harmony in her body and about calling forth the synthesis of p53 enzyme in every cell. She was dedicated to the practice, and she called me on the telephone several times to refine her meditations so they worked specifically for her. Imagery is a powerful tool when it is simple and personally meaningful.

Eventually, Anna came to my office for her sessions. Much of her stamina had returned; her spunk was in full display; and her questions were as astute as ever. Her head was wrapped in a bright scarf because she had progressively lost her hair from chemotherapy. This was evidence that both the cancerous and the healthy cells of her body were absorbing the powerful chemotherapy drugs. We worked with using the medications, both intravenous and oral, for her body's highest good, while continuing to fine-tune her balance and harmony, along with p53 visualizations.

Anna's tumor marker tests continue to show no tumor activity whatsoever, and her physician believes she will make a full recovery.

• • •

Cell-Level Healing in Practice

I've seen many cancer patients over the years. Some did not survive their disease. Some found the combination of meditation and medicine powerfully helpful, and they continued their spiritual practice long after they regained their health and there was no sign of cancer. A few, along with their alternative physician, chose to keep a close eye on the tumors while eschewing chemotherapy and explored acupuncture, herbs, supplements, and spiritual healing. A very few of those people had remarkable and complete recoveries. At this time in history, full recovery without medical intervention is rare. When clients combine spiritual and medical therapies, however, they report the best and most reliable results.

> *When clients combine spiritual and medical therapies, they report the best and most reliable results.*

Diabetes

Deep inside the pancreas—an elliptically shaped organ tucked neatly behind the stomach, sandwiched above the kidneys, and in front of the spine—thousands of cells churn out digestive enzymes. One part of the pancreas, small in size but enormous in impact on the body, contains the cells that make insulin. These cells are euphemistically named the *Islets of Langerhans* after the man who discovered them. They are filled with insulin, which they release into the bloodstream when it is needed, depending on the energy needs of the body. Among many important functions, insulin regulates glucose (simple sugar) metabolism. When the diet contains an excess of sugar and fatty foods, the need for insulin is high, and the cells may become exhausted from trying to keep up with the demand. At some point, the body no longer can respond and *insulin resistance* occurs; this condition is a forerunner of diabetes. An exhausted pancreas can make only a small amount of insulin, or no insulin at all, with serious side effects such as circulatory problems, blindness, and shock that may cause death. Although obesity and lack of exercise are risk factors in developing diabetes, the cause remains unknown. Recently, however, scientists postulate that diabetes may be a disease of the mitochondria.[2]

Healing meditations, a healthy lifestyle, exercise, and stress reduction have proven significantly helpful to many diabetics. However, they are not a substitution for medical treatment but rather complementary support.

In traditional spiritual lore, the *solar plexus*, located approximately in the pit of the stomach, is the site of personal power. The solar plexus exhibits the etheric color gold, representing the sun. Combining these ideas and images with biological information about the pancreas, the following meditations may help stabilize insulin levels and promote the highest degree of health possible. Feel free to adapt this exercise for your own needs.

> *In traditional spiritual lore, the* solar plexus,
> *located approximately in the pit of the stomach, is the site of personal power.*

2. Frederick H. Wilson et al., "A Cluster of Metabolic Defects Caused by Mutation in a Mitochondrial tRNA," *Science* 306 (2004): 1190–94.

BRIDGE TO HEALING

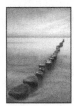

1. Imagine your solar plexus as a warm sun. Breathe into the central part of your body. Flood your midsection with the thought of warm, golden light.

2. Call forth your personal place in the world, your personal power; see yourself standing with golden light emanating in a spiral from your central core and surrounding your body. Deepen the reach of the golden light and your awareness into the cells of your pancreas.

3. Address the beta cells of the Islets of Langerhans, the cells busy making (or trying to make) insulin. Cheer them on; send them the support of your personal power. See them bathed in warm, golden light.

4. Imagine that you can journey even deeper: take your awareness into the mitochondria of the cells that produce insulin. Bring golden light to the mitochondria. Bring the consciousness of renewal, support, and new energy to any exhausted enzymes. Encourage the mitochondria to take in spiritual energy and integrate it for the work of producing physical energy for the body.

Emotional Issues

There are many kinds of emotional issues and a wide variety of therapeutic interventions. Let's look at some general categories of severity in emotional trauma and suggestions for the appropriate means of healing. Spiritual support can always be integrated with other interventions for healing.

> *Spiritual support can always be integrated*
> *with other interventions for healing.*

Severe emotional trauma

In cases of severe emotional trauma, medical and psychological treatment is crucial. In conjunction with a skilled therapist, spiritual support through your church, faith, meditation practice, or spiritual healer can assist in your recovery process. The cells of the brain, or entire portions of the brain, may be affected and blocked.

Calming yourself with deep meditative breath work can clear your mind and enable you to find the professional help you need. If the situation is in the distant past but continues to trouble you after you have exhausted therapeutic intervention, contact a spiritual healer or teacher, or your religious leader, for direct, personal assistance.

Moderate emotional upset

Upset often disrupts our steady sense of self and unseats us from our center in a way that may be distinctly felt in the body. The following meditations may be useful if an event or relationship is the root of emotional upset. This meditation will help you regain access to a rational and biochemically balanced state, where the situation and person(s) troubling you shift into less staggering proportions. The cells in your body will begin to receive messages of the return to equilibrium, and the biochemistry of high alert will shift back to normal.

BRIDGE TO HEALING

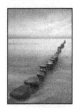

Here is an exercise for emotional issues:

1. Visualize bringing yourself back to a center within yourself, a calm and protected inner space where you are in touch with your spiritual resources.

2. Once centered, place yourself within the image of a personal safe place such as a garden or meadow that is protected by a gate, a wall, and guardian angels.

3. From that safe place, imagine the person or situation you are concerned about. Visualize spirals of clear light around them bringing blessing, harmony, and resolution. Do not try to make the outcome specific, but with trust, place the event or person(s) in the hands of the Divine Creator, Higher Power, God, or however you experience that Being or Creative Force.

4. Stay with the visualization until you feel a drop in tension, a relaxation into a less agitated or fearful state of mind. Continue to deepen the feelings of relaxation and the associated images with the intention to reach every cell of your body.

5. The cells of your body are now regaining their normal or "unflooded" state of physiology. The action portion of your cells, the endoplasmic reticulum, has shifted out of rapid production of "fight or flight" hormones. The communication system between cells is now also shifting out of the highly alert mode back toward normal.

6. When you feel the visualization is complete, see yourself alone in your special inner space. Surround yourself with glowing spirals of light. Actively accept blessing and renewal. Consciously depart from your inner space of safety, remembering that you can return anytime you wish.

Everyday emotional jolts

Watching the evening news can be an emotionally upsetting experience. How can you deal with the constant barrage of images and information that connect us with the traumas of the entire globe?

BRIDGE TO HEALING

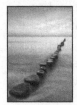

I use the following simple exercise for life's immediate and frequent challenges:

1. Awareness is the first part of the practice: notice when you are challenged by an image or information.

2. Assume that you can assist in some small way or you would not be touched by the situation.

3. Center and surround yourself with spirals of light. Then send a blessing of light to the troubled area. If there is something tangible that you can do, proceed to do it.

Many world issues are so large that we feel powerless. But we can trust that positive thoughts and light energy will help counterbalance the negativity surrounding us. Our cells go into stress mode when we are worried, which is damaging to health over the long term. Our internal chemistry changes, flooding the cells and the entire body with biochemicals that prepare us to fight or run from potential danger. Repeated events of this stress response eventually exhaust the body and damage our health. Rather than spending energy on the "what ifs" and "oh my goodnesses," concentrate on sending loving, positive energy for healing, resolution, and peace. Specific directives such as "Spouse, call me from the freeway!" or "Teen, if you don't do your homework, you will flunk!" are *not* recommended. These kinds of verbal communications belong in the practical world of direct, kinder, and actually effective speech.

> *Our cells go into stress mode when we are worried, which is damaging to health over the long term.*

Grief situations

The grieving process after the loss of a loved one begins with complete acceptance of your own feelings and state of being. You may need extra rest, long walks, seeing people, or not seeing people. Anticipate that each day will be different. When you are ready, seek others to talk with who have been through the grieving process and who are able to be with you and your range of emotions. When superficial platitudes leave your insides aching, release them as quickly as possible. Open yourself to receiving comfort from your spiritual resources in prayer, meditation, and silence. Prepare yourself for the possibility of your loved one's consciousness showing up in a dream or waking vision. Allow the comfort of visionary events without judgment or clinging. If no direct visions come, take heart from the stories of others such as those in Ray Moody's *Reunions*.[3]

A Personal Story

My mother died when I was twenty-five. Losing her was sudden, unexpected, and devastating. I was in graduate school and totally unprepared for such a loss. Every night for months, I woke myself crying in my dreams. There was no comfort to be found anywhere. People told me I should be brave, get over it, and move on with my life. I learned to put on a good front and bury my feelings of sadness and profound loss under the surface—way under the surface! Two years later, still having occasional dreams about her and waking up sobbing, I sought therapy. The process was immeasurably helpful, and I began to feel lighter, freer, and refocused on my busy and happy life.

After my daughter was born, during those long nights of rocking with an agitated newborn, I had a most unusual experience, espe-

3. Raymond Moody and Paul Perry, *Reunions: Visionary Encounters with Departed Loved Ones* (New York: Random House, Ivy Books, 1994).

cially for a down-to-earth scientist. (I had not yet received the call to healing.) I felt the spirit of my mother place her arms around me and the baby as I sat in the rocking chair. She stayed with us until the baby was asleep again. I knew it was my mother because her energy and her sweet touch were unmistakable. I had never imagined that something like this could happen, and it was not a one-time-only event. She came to us in spirit many times. I could not force this experience; no particular thought or desire brought her to us, but I recognized her presence instantly.

$$\bullet \quad \bullet \quad \bullet$$

When you are grieving, long after the hot casseroles from the neighbors are consumed, long after the wise and seasoned therapist can lead you safely through the intense emotions of grief, comfort can come. The unexpected visitation, a spiritual blessing, or a vision may touch you with ineffable grace and unshakable faith. All of the cells in your body will respond, culminating in 100 trillion sighs of exceptional peace.

Medication

Most of us, at some unexpected and unwelcome time, will require medication that we would rather not need to take. From a strong anti-inflammatory for plantar fasciitis to prednisone for bee stings to chemotherapy for cancer treatment, the arsenal of strong medicines developed by modern science can frighten the formerly healthy. The need for pharmaceutical drugs is particularly challenging for those of us who eat organic foods and drink water as free of pollutants and contaminant chemicals as possible. We look for alternatives to allopathic medicines.

The sense of failure haunts a formerly well person: "What did I do wrong? How can I correct my thoughts or actions to make this go away?" Every pill or intravenous treatment becomes a reminder of the disappointment in oneself, in one's associates, or in God. Worse than a reminder, many people fight medication with moments of anger and resentment, even while swallowing the prescription. Evelyn's situation is a good example:

• • •

Evelyn had been healthy all her life. Robustly healthy! How could the diagnosis of ovarian cancer possibly be true when she felt good, looked great, and was embarking on such a wonderful time in her life of companionship, travel, and retirement ease? The confusion around her made accepting the diagnosis even more difficult. Not until surgery revealed masses of inoperable tumors metastasized throughout her abdomen and in her bones did she really believe the doctor's words. Deciding to accept chemotherapy was another hurdle of immense proportion, and she nearly refused. When I was called to her bedside, she was slowly coming back to herself after surgery, but she was in the throes of making that important decision about chemotherapy.

How did we get to the place of considering the best of allopathic medicine to be bad for us? Certainly there are the horror stories of misdiagnoses, of medicines that had harmful effects, of the wrong solution being put in a patient's intravenous. These errors are highlighted, but the thousands of good treatments are not mentioned. Clearly, we all need advocates, questions, and caution about any treatment.

Evelyn had completed her "homework" on the various issues related to having cancer, yet she anguished over taking chemotherapy and the other medications necessary to make her more comfortable or prevent nausea. Our discussions focused on the scary stories stuck in her mind that continued to create fear. One common belief among the holistically minded is that any medication, and chemotherapy in particular, hurts the immune system and actually prevents the body from healing. Evelyn and I discussed her options, settled on a rational plan, and then plunged much deeper into our work. That deeper work gave Evelyn new tools to enhance her comfort and, hopefully, the efficacy of the medication. Her treatment was successful, and she is now in remission.

• • •

If you are experiencing illness and your doctor prescribes medication, the following steps can be taken, which can be adapted according to your personal situation:

1. Make sure you have the best information possible from medical science. After a second opinion, when you feel you have all the data you need, proceed to the next step.

2. Approach any medical procedure or medication with relaxed confidence that you have made a good decision for yourself under the given circumstances.

3. Quell the opposing opinions within yourself, as if bringing two (or more) warring parties together at a mediation table. Ambivalence is one thing, but internal war is truly self-destructive. Bless the medications and ask that they do the work intended for your body's healing and the very best possible outcome.

4. As you swallow your pills, welcome them into your body as a healing potion.

> *Approach any medical procedure or medication with relaxed confidence that you have made a good decision for yourself under the given circumstances.*

5. If you are receiving chemotherapy by intravenous drip, as the equipment is being set up, take those moments to bless the medicine for its best work in your body. Similarly, with radiation, bless the energy that is about to be beamed into your tissues. Relax and focus on the treatment as beneficial.

6. Ask that the chemo, radiation, or other medication easily find the cells that need to recycle: the cancer cells whose molecules can then be discarded as waste or used by your body for building normal cells. In turn, ask that the healthy cells of your body be minimally affected and that side effects be as slight as possible.

7. Once again, as the treatment begins or the pill is swallowed, relax into some moments of meditation of welcome in your body of the wonder of medical science and its healing properties as needed for your specific situation.

Menopause

Much good material has been written about menopause, including the various opinions about supplemental hormone treatment for symptoms such as hot flashes and night sweats. Hormone replacement therapy (HRT) is helpful beyond imagination for some women. A physician told me that patients have demanded continued access to HRT with a vehemence quite unexpected. For others, the side effects make HRT unpleasant and undesirable. I found myself a disappointed and unhappy member of this second category. Even with HRT, my symptoms went unabated; I experienced rampant night sweats and those strange sensations of rising heat in my neck. It felt like my entire body was on fire.

Out of desperation, having tried acupuncture, herbs, estrogen, progesterone in pill and cream form, and various vitamins, I sat down to *listen* to my body. The direction my body was taking—reducing hormonal levels and the shutting down of fertility cycles—was the normal pattern of my biology. When my hormone levels dropped too abruptly, however, symptoms would appear. This was my understanding from listening to my body. The next step was to use this information to ameliorate the hot flashes and sweating. That would test the efficacy of my ideas immediately.

What could I do to slow the process when my hormonal levels were dropping too fast? The need was not for buckets of hormones but for only a few additional molecules. Eventually, I was able to stop a hot flash before it progressed any further by using visualizations. If a hot flash was well underway, it would dissipate immediately. You can try this yourself:

BRIDGE TO HEALING

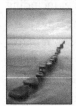

When you begin to feel a hot flash starting, stop whatever you are doing and take a minute to tune in to your body. Imagine that you can connect with all of the hormone-producing locations in your body and communicate with them. Ask your body to produce a few more molecules of either estrogen or progesterone, whichever is most needed to stop the hot flash or night sweats.

Perhaps it was only my ability to relax that was effective, or maybe, just maybe, I was able to shift my body's comfort levels with a conscious intention for balance and peace. Could it be that, as my intention deepened into a focus on the cells responsible for producing the molecules involved, I was actually able to change the hormonal environment of my blood?

Many of my clients have found this technique to be as effective for them as it was for me. Others discovered that using HRT worked better. For some, the combination of both medical and mental intervention eased the way through this powerful change of life. Menopause is, after all, transformation into a truly powerful part of our feminine selves.

Multiple Sclerosis

Maureen Manley loves riding a bicycle. She remembers vividly her first bike, a "sissy" bike: "It was canary yellow, had a long banana-shaped and hideously flowered seat, tassels on the sissy handle-bars, and skinny tires with fenders."

Her parents realized right away that Maureen was aghast with the look of her new bike, even at the age of ten, so they helped transform the sissy bike into a black "machine" with a slick racing seat; thick, knobby tires with no fenders; and black racing cross bars with no tassels. Every new boy in the neighborhood was initiated by the other guys by being set up to race her—and lose.

Lots of road, lots of bikes, and lots of growing up from that first tasseled two-wheeler culminated in the elite athlete: Maureen Manley, member of the U.S. Cycling Team, a national record setter, holder of two national championships among other medals, and many championship awards. As a result, she loves all aspects of the sport: peak physical fitness, including hundreds of hours of training, finely honed skill, and well-engineered bicycle equipment. Maureen is smart. She has the kind of brain power required for racing strategy, the steady nerves to ride very fast in tight formation, and the gumption to enjoy the hair-breadth precision required of a world-class rider.

In the tradition of competitive athletes, Maureen was able to ride past pain. When she began to experience uncanny fatigue and mildly blurred vision, she attributed it to over-training. She was sure these symptoms were something she could ride through and past. Setting her steely mind on the road ahead, her body usually performed regardless of scrapes, aches, or throbbing muscles. In 1991, while riding with the U.S. Women's Team on the first stage of the Tour de France (Tour Feminin for women), her mind was on the hill climb that late August day. Then she realized something was wrong. Her legs were on fire with the effort as she pushed her body, and she lunged up off the bicycle seat to get more push to the pedals.

"The harder I rode the climb, the worse my vision got. When I crashed at the top of the hill, my vision had blurred so much that I rode my bike off the road and crashed."

It was neither a freak incident nor a temporary attack of the flu. The doctor later confirmed a diagnosis of multiple sclerosis (MS).

MS is a disease of the brain, spinal cord, and optic nerve that is not associated with an infection, nor is it contagious. MS is considered to be an autoimmune disease, which means the body attacks its own tissues and destroys its own cells. The complicated events leading to cell degeneration are unknown. What is known is that nearly twice as many women are affected as men, and certain geographic locations have a higher incidence than others. The progression of MS is carefully charted and described according to symptoms, with the different forms of MS labeled as relapsing-remitting, primary-progressive, secondary-progressive, and progressive-relapsing.

At the cellular level, the affected nerve cells in the central nervous system (CNS) lose their protective myelin sheath. Myelin wraps around the process of nerve cells, their axons, and is composed of a small amount of protein (20 percent). Fatty tissue or lipid molecules make up the other 80 percent. Specialized cells in the CNS called *oligodendrocytes* have long arms that lend structural support to the axons of several nerves and produce myelin wherever they touch the nerves. Myelin is crucial for the transmission of messages along nerve cells, because it insulates the nerves and allows a speedy and accurate message to travel to its destination: the next nerve cell in the relay sequence that will eventually tell a muscle when to contract. The damaging effects of MS may make walking difficult or impossible, or impair bladder function.

Maureen had all of the primary symptoms of MS: severe impairment in muscle function, fatigue, and problems with vision. Thus began a different kind of journey—one requiring fitness, attention, skill, and focus on the immediate "road" conditions while walking with a cane and enduring erratically undependable eyesight. Maureen proceeded through medical assessment and treatment. Availing herself of steroid treatment, she participated fully in the latest medications that her doctor prescribed.

Maureen also branched out to alternative therapies when she had exhausted what allopathic medicine had to offer, including nutritional regimens, vitamin supplements, Reiki, psychotherapy, massage; you name it, she tried it.

When she came to me in 1999, eight years after the onset of MS, she had already recovered considerably. Referred by a trusted friend and instructor, Maureen was, understandably, skeptical. Many therapies and therapists had promised cures. Some helped, some made her worse, and some were ineffective regardless of the effort involved. In spite of her past disappointments, Maureen plunged into exploring what we could achieve together.

During her first visit, we discussed what she had already accomplished: her eyes worked fine, most of the time, and she was able to walk without a cane, although she was a bit unsteady. Maureen worked out at a gym and rode a stationary bicycle. Unable to ride her bike outside on a road, and certainly not in a group with friends or competitors, a major aspect of her delight and verve of life seemed gone forever.

In her own words, Maureen experienced profound healing from our work, including more stability in her vision, less fatigue, stronger legs, and steadier overall body function.

"I was surprised and amazed as my body responded to the work," she said. "I was surprised at what my body was capable of doing. I experienced subtle changes in energy that translated into improved ability after the session."

Maureen's unstoppable spirit, our healing work, and the best of medical science and pharmaceuticals eventually enabled Maureen to ride the road again and also to compete. She has ridden several races, a time trial, and several organized group rides. One was the 2005 Seattle to Portland, a 180-mile event in one day. Another, in 2005, was the 150-mile MS fund-raising ride in two days, with Maureen delivering a keynote address after the first day's ride. She is thrilled with her new capacities and ability to return to competitive cycling.

"With increased life and energy in my body, I am not going backwards with the disease. I am going forward in my life," she said.

As with my other clients, my work with Maureen includes energy healing and spiritual support, which alleviate the enormous fear of an uncertain future: "Will my body stabilize or slowly worsen and then cataclysmically deteriorate?" The stress of the unknown creates its own health challenges. Recognizing and naming the fear places it out in the open. Then we can imagine bundling up our particular fears and lifting them into the hands of the Universe. The biggest challenge is to trust life energy and your spiritual connection enough to relax and let the healing happen.

> *The biggest challenge is to trust life energy*
> *and your spiritual connection enough to*
> *relax and let the healing happen.*

BRIDGE TO HEALING

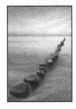

This meditation is specifically for MS:

1. *Stop the damage to brain cells.* Imagine a wave of cool energy moving into the top of your head and passing all the way down through your body. Imagine that the coolness soothes and stops any progression of nerve damage. Use the words "Healing energy" as a mantra with each in-breath. As you breathe out, send the image "Stabilize" to all your nerves. Do seven rounds of this practice twice a day.

2. *Clean up the damaged areas.* Ask the wise cells of the central nervous system, which have the job of cleaning up debris (astrocytes and microglia), to gently remove scar tissue. Using a wave of energy, imagine loosening the tight zipper of the lesions to give space for new life to course throughout. Ask the oligodendrocytes

to wrap their snug spiral blanket around the nerve cells. See them spinning their fine work, creating insulation, and thereby promoting the return to full nerve function.

3. *Connect brain to peripheral nerves.* Envision gently moving energy from one nerve cell in the brain to another, and then to a peripheral nerve that, in turn, connects with an affected muscle. Create an image of the flow of information moving smoothly from brain to spinal cord, and then to muscle—and the muscle working properly.

Surgery

Surgeons are perhaps the most skillful people on planet Earth. They have to be smart, have terrific hand-eye coordination, and be born with nerves of steel. If you need surgery, you want a well-trained, exceedingly experienced, alert, and focused doctor. Find a competent surgeon and medical team you can trust.

The material in this section consists of two parts: how to prepare yourself for surgery and how to have advocates work for you. These suggestions come from my experience in working with people before surgery, immediately after surgery, and during recovery after leaving the hospital. Hundreds of clients have proven the efficacy of these methods.

Preparing yourself

Having exhausted all other routes of healing, know that surgery is the best healing modality for you, given the circumstances.

Accept and welcome the surgery and the accompanying medications as healing modalities that will ultimately give you back the part of your life that is now compromised by disease. When you take medications, pause and bless them to do their work in your body.

Working with your advocates

Meet with your family and friends before the surgery. Have them join you for a few hours one evening. They need to know each other and establish a phone or e-mail link. One person should become the liaison with your medical team and be listed in your chart as having the authority to access your records (if you want this). This person can call the hospital to receive updates on your condition and relay the information to your other advocates.

Have someone with you when you talk to the doctor before your surgery. Ask this particular advocate to take notes and to remind you of questions you may have forgotten to ask.

Ask a group of family and friends to meditate or pray for you during the five days prior to the surgery, during the surgery, and for five days afterwards.

Have someone with you when you talk to the doctor before your surgery.

Develop a schedule so that one or two advocates are with you during the first twenty-four to thirty-six hours after surgery. They can help by managing the number of visitors, answering the phone until you want to do it yourself, and communicating with the nursing staff if you need something. You are not expected to be a social whiz after surgery, so don't try to have brilliant conversations and exhaust yourself.

Your advocates are also important as spiritual resources. Ask them to meditate or pray for you around these specific issues:

- Ask that your body will be fully ready for the surgery, bleeding will be minimal, the site of surgery will be easy for the surgeon to access, and your body will accept the procedure being done. For example, if there is a tumor, ask that all the cells be clustered together, making them easy to remove.

- Ask that the medical team is rested and totally focused so they can do their best. Surround the surgeon, the anesthesiologist, and all of the surgical staff with light and support.

Healing at an Even Deeper Level

Adrian had a serious attack of appendicitis when she was seven years old. Her family, particularly her father, did not believe in conventional medicine, physicians, or hospitals, and he tried other means to help his seriously ill daughter—primarily prayer. At death's doorway, and against the edicts of her father, Adrian was finally rushed to a hospital where she needed painful and invasive procedures to clean up the extensive infection in her abdomen. The initial surgery to remove her appendix was the least of her agonizing treatments.

She came to me in her late forties, after years of extensive therapy, which had helped her cope with the trauma of her early experience. But she wanted more. She wanted a relaxed and natural way of being in the world, not tight and timid as she had thought was necessary. Why did she choose to try a spiritual healer, particularly with her early history of religious belief that prevented her from necessary medical assistance? Adrian was referred by one of her very dear friends, who had been a long-term client of mine, and who had healed from significant childhood trauma. Although Adrian was understandably tentative about working with me, she had seen the benefits for her friend.

Perhaps the fact that I do not consider spiritual healing as a stand-alone path to health helped Adrian resolve her "either/or" arguments about medicine and spirituality. I believe we all need medical help from time to time, including preventive checkups to confirm that we continue to be healthy. Medicine and spirituality *can* be integrated. We can enrich our lives and our health by once again linking a spiritual dimension as part of our lifestyle. The bridge from soul to cell can also become a bridge between spirituality and medicine.

Medicine and spirituality can *be integrated.*

In general, Adrian found that the principles of appreciation, clearing blockages, Flow, and Cell-Level Healing improved her sense of well-being. These practices supported her exploration into career choices she had dreamed about but did not have the self-assurance to pursue. The work helped her learn to deal with authoritarian personalities without losing her confidence. She began to trust her natural spirituality and healing ability. Perhaps the work reached those memory cells that had been frozen in time and fear.

Adrian called me and asked for an appointment with the most excitement I had ever heard in her voice. We met and she spoke about dreams she had not previously mentioned.

"I've had a recurring dream for almost thirty years—since I was a teenager. In the dream I am being chased by three men. All of them look alike and they want to kill me. It is so horrible and terrifying. I run and run, but they eventually catch me. Just at the moment I am about to die, I wake up. I've had times when I stayed up all night to avoid having this dream.

"It had been a while since I had one of these dreams, until last week. However, the setting of this dream was a bit different. Rather than there being only myself and three assailants, I dreamed that I was surrounded by a small army of helpers, and we were being attacked by an evil army. I had a map in my hand, and I was sending parts of my army to various places in attempting to lay out some strategy. Suddenly you [Joyce] appeared and looked at the map. You took it from my hands and said that you didn't like this at all. When you crumpled up the map and threw it away, all the armies disappeared! I woke up happy, not at all scared, and amazed that my dream had changed so much."

This was not Adrian's really good dream, however. It gets better!

"Two nights later, I was back in the army dream, just as before.

"I had the map in my hand and was hurriedly planning my strategy. Then I spoke, saying, 'I don't like this!' and I crumpled up the map and threw it away—myself."

I was thrilled that Adrian could take her healing deep into the memory cells of her subconscious mind and create a scenario of such strength that she stepped into her personal power. Our spiritual work had reached her deepest places of trauma, freeing her from three decades of dreamtime terror.

Conclusion

One of my grandfathers had a stroke at age sixty-two, and he was thought to have only a short time to live. In fact, he recovered, outlived his wife, bowled in a league, and planted summer gardens for several widows in his hometown of Camas, Washington, at ninety-five. He died peacefully at ninety-eight after a fourteen-day bout with a respiratory infection.

One of my best friends, a woman who is always trim, exercises regularly, and eats more vegetables than the entire neighborhood, had a sudden onset of non-Hodgkin's lymphoma. Not one but certainly two if not three different types of lymphoma pushed her body close to death. Experimental treatment followed by a stem cell transplant saved her life. A team of friends, including me, met each week during her months in the hospital to pray for her recovery. Six years later, she remains robustly healthy, still eating vegetables, exercising, and making a difference in our community.

For all of us, uncertainty is a reality of human life, but if we live in apprehension of accidents or illness we surrender part of our lifetime to fear. We can, instead, look directly at our concerns, gather them, and release them into the Universe, to a Higher Source. Truly, the biggest challenge is to trust enough to relax fully into life.

8

The Ultimate Healing Bridge

**Although I was classically trained
in biology, as a doctoral student in biophysics,
I was immersed in the study of physics, much to my chagrin.**
As a biologist I was trained in direct observation, often by looking into one or several types of microscopes. Not having had previous graduate-level training in physics, I was amazed to discover that, rather than viewing the world by observation, physicists envision the universe in elegant equations. One of the tests I was required to pass was to be able to write all of the essential equations as to how the universe works on a 3 x 5 card and explain the full and profound meaning of each one. This is called *reductionist science* for a very good and obvious reason.

The dimension of time was not one of those mathematical wonders on our cards. In fact, physicists go to great lengths to cancel out "t," because it messes up most of the solutions to their elegant equations. Time is not steady, especially in quantum mechanics; it varies with changes in other qualities, such as speed. As modern, or quantum, physics has seeped into the culture and trendy thinking, the problem of time has been handled as an illusion. By doing so, the world and all of us in it have become illusions.

Cell-Level Healing

Without the help of science, many ancient mystical traditions had already decided that life on earth is an illusion, but when modern physics and spirituality came together, the whole of existence, including time, advanced into the realm of illusion.

This is truly an enigma for a biologist. Physical life in the body, so wondrously structured, is dependent on time. Cell events occur in swift packets of time; the biochemistry of metabolism speeds along in nanoseconds or picoseconds. Elaborate codes embedded in the DNA determine how long the cells of each tissue and organ will live. Special enzymes cause cells to die early if the codes that determine the time of replication are misread or overlooked. To a biological system, time is of the essence—literally, it is essential. Time makes life possible.

Time factors control your own experience every day. The cycles of rest, sleep, waking, eating, working, and recreation all involve time. Our perception of time can shift and change with circumstances. For a major-league baseball player facing a 95-mph, four-seam fastball, time seems to slow down. The ball looks like a blur to those watching from the stands, but to the player, including the all-time hitting master Ichiro (Seattle Mariners, 2004), it is visible and hittable. Time seems to disappear when you are engaged in an activity that takes all of your focus. You either have all the time you need, or you don't notice how much time has transpired. Your cells, however, have automatically continued the activities of life without your attention—and without a clock.

Our perception of time may change, but a level of biological reality persists. I propose that we no longer dismiss our bodies, our lives, as illusions or physical spaces beyond our reach, but rather, embrace them as sacred dimensions. In that embrace, we enhance our lives, value our environment, and use our time well.

Many spiritually minded people ignore or deny illness or injury, especially the early signals that something in the body is "not right." Faulty thinking chimes in and they tell themselves, "It's just an illusion. Envision yourself beyond this ache, this pain, this symptom." While ignoring the problem, the risk of the condition worsening continues. Over and over again, early detection and medical treatment prove to offer the best chance for recovery.

How a person understands reality and illusion influences how they use healing energy. Translating spiritual blessing to the body—the Flow from Soul to Cell—is the interface between the etheric and the material world. Like the interface of ocean and land, although the medium is different, liquid interfaces with solid, and both are real.

If you hold the spiritual dimension and the physical dimension at a point of tension, you may find the awareness of the two pushing each other back and forth. At this tension point, however, you can receive the blessings of spiritual awareness and healing, while at the same time, an appreciation of the physical world allows you to use science to the fullest. If you can see your body as an expression of the sacred while at the same time recognizing its purely physical properties and needs, then you are well equipped to navigate your life and its challenges with access to the best resources of both realities.

> *If you hold the spiritual dimension and the physical dimension at a point of tension, you may find the awareness of the two pushing each other back and forth.*

Spirituality and Death

Before my near-death experience, I thought there was no afterlife and, consequently, no continuation of consciousness. In my view, death was total, complete, and utterly final. Much to my surprise and joy, after my near-death experience the notion of continuation of consciousness became an unshakable reality. It was not an abstract idea or a passage in a book but an experience of the fabulous riches of total peace and belonging that eased my concerns about death. Actually, more than easing my concerns, my fear of death left and has not returned. Part of my work as a healer includes being called by families to the bedside of their dying loved ones. Odd as it may sound, helping someone find peace through prayer and meditation as they enter the afterlife is profoundly intense and strangely joyful.

Staying centered in the hope of a conscious, good death is a valuable endeavor for anyone, and conversations with a counselor, pastor, or family member can be quite helpful. The closer death comes, the more the universal experience of being welcomed to the other side increases. Materialism, status, and defended beliefs drop away. We enter the world naked, and we leave our body without credentials, bank accounts, or designer jeans.

The process of leaving the physical body has been well described in writings such as Sherwin B. Nuland's *How We Die: Reflections on Life's Final Chapter* and Elisabeth Kübler-Ross's *On Death and Dying*.[1] Many religions describe the soul leaving the body and hold

1. Sherwin B. Nuland, *How We Die: Reflections on Life's Final Chapter* (New York: Vintage, Anchor, 1995); Elisabeth Kübler-Ross, *On Death and Dying* (New York: Scribner, 1997).

different beliefs about intermediate states of being, journeys down tunnels, across rivers, on paths in the jungle, and out across an expanse of emptiness. My own experiences at the bedside are not gauged by a particular belief system but are offered here from personal observation.

When a patient is in a coma, with all of their vital signs still functioning, and their soul departs, the feeling in the room changes. The person looks different in a manner difficult to describe. Usually the final signs of death—heart stopped and no respiration—occur within ten to thirty minutes after the mysterious departure of the soul. The person's consciousness may remain near the body for some time, but frequently, and especially with preparation, the soul takes immediate flight to the safety of the beyond: Heaven, Heart of God, Universe, Creator, or luminous emptiness—however you may think of the afterlife.

Two general principles have emerged from my work with people approaching and completing this transition between the physical and spiritual realms:

The fear of death reduces the fullness of life and holds part of us captive.
and
When we face and overcome our fear of death,
we can live in a new dimension of ease, clarity, and vitality.

Let me illustrate my understanding of the bridge that overcomes the fear of death, allows a new appreciation and fullness of life, and can support us in our own death or help us to compassionately assist others at their time of crossing over.

Cell-Level Healing

One of the key elements of training for indigenous healers in remote (or not-so-remote, anymore) parts of the world is personally facing death. The intent is to conquer this ultimate fear and then be able to walk between the worlds of physical and purely spiritual realities. Most of these training events are overwhelmingly fearsome. In Bali, an aspiring healer may be taken by the teacher to a specific temple situated on an oceanside rocky outcrop of land that is accessible only during low tide. The initiate is left there to spend the night without shelter, food, or water. Alone in the open air, as the tide slips around the temple perched on rock, night settles in with unabated inky darkness. The waves crash all around the initiate and cobras emerge from their underground dens to investigate the intruder. The *only* way to survive this ordeal is to sit in the stillness of meditation with no fear. Perhaps you can imagine my gratitude that my tests, arduous enough for me, did not include this particular one.

If the healer is alive and sane when the tidal waters recede, the initiation is considered complete and successful. Is there any doubt why shamans and indigenous healers are so respected in their communities? At work in their villages, these healers are expected to bridge between worlds in order to obtain information for the family from the spirit realms. Perhaps there is an herb, a source of healing water, a ritual, or advice on an emotional issue that could help bring peace to the troubled individual. On occasion, the healing unexpectedly reaches into the cells of the body and brings remarkable physical healing. My ten years of study, during six trips to Bali, provided me with an understanding of the value of carefully crossing the chasm between heaven and earth—and between meditative states of consciousness and ordinary perception.

The Ultimate Healing Bridge

The wisdom of Jero Mangku Sri Kandi, my Balinese teacher and mentor, transcended cultural rituals and beliefs. She was a master healer with great skill in linking dimensions of consciousness. Over a decade of experiencing her rigorous tests, her implacable demeanor, and her profoundly loving spiritual connection, she taught me to safely and reliable embrace a greater reality beyond the material world.

Although I was not required to endure an overnight with cobras, in one of our ceremonies on the east coast of Bali, Jero Mangku directed me to sit in a certain place at a remote temple. Then she walked ahead three or four feet and began chanting. To my shocked amazement I was sitting at the entrance to a heavily populated and busy red-ant hill. These fire ants, infamous for their nasty bite, were running about, all over the place. My attention, however, came back immediately to the sound of Jero Mangku's chanting, and I entered a blissful state of mind. In twenty sweaty (a side effect of the weather, not the ants) but peaceful minutes the ants went about their own business. Not one bit me! Certainly one of her most memorable tests, Jero Mangku repeatedly placed me in situations that required the qualities of focus, fearlessness, and compassion.

I have since learned to apply in my work as a healer the more than thirty conscious passages Jero safely facilitated for me. These practices provide information for my clients that can only be perceived during altered states of consciousness so deep that they almost approach a deathlike state. The knowledge I gained from working with Jero has helped me as a healer in my own culture, without the necessity of reproducing Balinese temples, clouds of incense, a gamelan orchestra, or a startling chant.

• • •

Cell-Level Healing

Carl was only forty years old when he was diagnosed with cancer. He had sought medical assistance after the pain became unbearable. I was called by his wife to his bedside at a hospice center attached to a local hospital. My first meeting with Carl was upbeat and interspersed with visitors coming to cheer him. Carl's bedside was a social event. He was not ready to die, although his tumors had massive metastases and his prognosis held no promise of recovery. Over weeks of short visits, usually interrupted by his many friends, family, and colleagues, the end approached. No longer besieged with visitors, only his wife came to the hospice unit to see Carl. He was sleeping more and more, and his breathing was intermittent and labored. When Carl's breath repeatedly stopped, his wife hoped each time that it was his final rest and relief from intense suffering. Sadly, he would shudder back to life, appearing terrified.

At this point, I was called. With both his wife and myself at his bedside, I synchronized my breath and awareness with his. I journeyed with him into the altered states of consciousness I had learned to navigate safely under Jero Mangku's tutelage. I saw fearsome images looming before him and understood why he had jammed back into his body. In seeing what he saw, I could speak quietly to him, guiding him past the frightening illusions. I paused with him and encouraged him to move steadily toward the light beyond all the apparitions. The energy from this extraordinary light communicated Divine Love and welcome, we proceeded until he finally broke completely free from his body and soared toward the light. Tremendous peace pervaded the room. Carl's wife acknowledged that he was gone, free, and blissfully at peace, and then we wept together, almost in joy.

• • •

Choosing to die at home, Sarah had left the hospital with all of her treatment completed and only pain management to help her during her transition. Meeting her for the first time at her home, I was directed to her bedroom, a small space with a futon bed, a high window, and respectfully quiet roommates. As I sat beside her, silently meditating, she seemed to slip into a comalike state. However, there was no sense of her life being at an end. No death energy lingered around her. I simply tracked her while staying fully grounded in present time and space. It seemed that my work was to provide an anchor for her return. After nearly an hour, she opened her eyes and excitedly told me about her vision. She had seen a glorious light. She described a beautiful place where she felt totally whole. Sarah virtually glowed with a perceptible light of her own as we spoke.

When I returned a week later, she looked much better, and she was even able to walk a bit. We went ahead with another healing session. Similar to the first session, Sarah found that place of beauty and healing, returning with more amazing stories of light and peace and glowing with an even more strongly emerging radiance. Sarah said she felt markedly better. Eventually she recovered significantly, as her journeys to the other side seemed to fill her with healing energy. She eventually died eight months later, but she had used the extra time extremely well. She found a sustained sense of peace, viewed her life with new awareness and appreciation, and accepted loving care from her formerly estranged family. Although not a cure, our work together was profoundly healing.

When assisting a person who may appear to be dying, energy from the other side may actually be physically healing. Not fearing the journey beyond this material reality allows us to gather healing energy for physical life. We do return easily, unless it is truly our time to make our transition. Each morning in my own meditations, I envision a bridge to the other side and ask to cross it in order to bask in the luminous energy and then return to my day's work. Sometimes it looks like a mossy footbridge on a mountain trail. At other times it stretches across the sky with rainbow colors. My sense of connection and being "at home" both in my body and the universe are enhanced with each meditative session. In working with others, I often feel as if I have one foot here and one foot on the other side. The clarity of insight and palpable touch of healing energy are strongest at those times. Over the years, the gap between this side and the other has shortened, and the bridge is not as vast as it once was.

> *When assisting a person who may appear to be dying, energy from the other side may actually be physically healing.*

May your own practice of gratitude, clearing, focus, and Cell-Level Healing create your own bridge to connect Soul to Cell and back again, thereby extinguishing any fear of death. May your experiences be safe and blessed, and may they sustain you in all your endeavors.

Appendix

**From the cloistered halls of academic laboratories to
the *Wall Street Journal* and the *Denver Post*, brain research
has entered an entirely new field of interest and understanding.**
This newly discovered ability of the brain to change both function
and structure in response to training is called neuroplasticity. One
of the primary tools of study is electroencephalographic (EEG)
recording of brainwave activity.

The malleability of our brains has led researchers to record brain
dexterity during advanced meditation, and the findings have gener-
ated surprising information and intriguing applications to each of us
for health. "What we found is that the longtime practitioners showed
brain activation on a scale we have never seen before," said Richard
Davidson, a neuroscientist at the University of Wisconsin's W. M. Keck
Laboratory for Functional Brain Imaging and Behavior.[1]

Building evidence shows the ability of our brain to adapt, with
training, to positive patterns that include feelings of well-being,
decreased anxiety, improved immune function, and even abiding
happiness and bliss. When engaged in meditation over a long period

1. Marc Kaufman, "Meditation Gives Brain a Charge, Study Finds," 3 January
2005, *www.washingtonpost.com*.

of time, the brain shows powerful bursts of specific activity and unusual coordination or synchrony.

"Davidson charted the normal, emotional states in the brains of 150 people, including Buddhist monk, Ricard. Most people fell into the middle ground between positive and negative emotions. But Ricard, who had been deeply meditating on compassion when his brain was scanned, nearly soared off the chart of positive emotions—the highest level of happiness ever documented."[2]

Before the current wave of interest, curiosity led Juan Acosta-Urquidi, Ph.D., and myself to test my brain activity in 2002 while in meditation and sending healing energy to someone three thousand miles away. My subjective experience during meditation was that of entering a deep state of exquisite oneness. Our preliminary data indicated that the subjective sense of oneness coincided with strong delta power. Bursts of delta and beta occurred as I was focused on sending healing energy. My alpha waves also increased.

Three years later, in July 2005, I was invited to Dr. Akio Mori's laboratory at Nihon University in Tokyo, Japan, to be filmed for a documentary that aired on Nokia TV, Channel 4, in Japan on August 8, 2005. Dr. Mori, a venerated professor of neurology, is a leading research scientist in the field of brain mapping. His comments on my 128-sensor EEG data, which was gathered while I sent healing to a cancer patient, were that I exhibited an extraordinary level of concentration and unusual activity in the left prefrontal cortex: the site of happiness. My internal sense of happiness while doing this work

2. Colleen O'Conner, "Willing Your Way to Happiness," 4 June 2006, *www.denverpost.com.*

is not the same as finding a bargain at the half-yearly shoe sale but of being in a state of nearly indescribable bliss. It is a kind of well-being that comes from the repeated experience of helping someone through the skillful focus of healing energy.

In June 2006, Dr. Acosta-Urquidi and a portable EEG device recorded my brain activity during meditation and while working on two clients sitting about six feet in front of me. The data generally resembled our 2002 scans but showed even higher levels of focused delta waves, peaks of beta, and increased alpha during healing. Also notable were new indications of high-frequency gamma brainwaves along with high levels of coordinated brain activity. For more information on gamma synchrony, see Antoine Lutz, L. L. Greischar, N. B. Rawlings, M. Ricard, and R. J. Davidson, "Long-term Meditators Self-induce High-amplitude Gamma Synchrony during Mental Practice," *Proceedings of the National Academy of Sciences* 101, no. 46 (2004): 16369–73.

The EEG equipment that Dr. Acosta-Urquidi used was conventional: a Mitsar Instrument (St. Petersburg, Russia) employing a 19-channel electrocap hookup, 10-20 International system, and referential linked ears montage. Raw data was analyzed to yield power-frequency spectra and topographic brain maps (QEEG). For additional information on his work, see J. Acosta-Urquidi, "Brainwaves and Heartwaves: Psychophysiological and Spiritual Dimensions of Energy Healing," *Journal of Alternative and Complementary Medicine* 10, no. 4 (2004): 728.

Appendix

Photography Credits

The publisher gratefully acknowledges and thanks the following for permission to use previously published photographs:

49. Hawkes, Joyce W. "The Effects of Petroleum Hydrocarbons on Fish: Morphological Changes." In *Proceedings of a Symposium of Fate and Effects of Petroleum Hydrocarbons in Marine Ecosystems and Organisms.* Edited by D. A. Wolfe. New York: Pergamon Press, 1977, 115–68.

50. Hawkes, J. W., and C. M. Stehr. "Ultrastructural Studies of Marine Organisms: A Manual of Techniques and Applications." *Electron Optics Bulletin* 118 (1982): 15–20.

51. Hawkes, J. W. "The Structure of Fish Skin. II. The Chromatophore Unit." *Cell and Tissue Research* 149 (1974): 159–74.

52. Top: Hawkes, J. W., 1974, unpublished data; bottom: Hawkes, J. W., 1974, unpublished data.

53. Hawkes, J. W. "The Effects of Xenobiotics on Fish Tissues: Morphological Studies." *Federation Proceedings* 39, no. 14 (1980): 3230–36.

54. Hawkes, J. W., 1976, unpublished data.

58. Hawkes, J. W. "The Structure of Fish Skin. III. The Chromatophore Unit of Albinistic Rainbow Trout (*Salmo gairdneri*)." *Scanning Electron Microscopy* 4 (1982): 1725–30.

62. Spiral Galaxy M101 from *www.hubblesite.org/gallery/album/galaxy_collection/pr2006010a/*.

75. Mori, Akio, July 2005. Dr. Hawkes tested in Dr. Akio Mori's Laboratory at Nihon University in Tokyo, Japan. Documentary aired on Nokia TV, Channel 4, in Japan on August 8, 2005.

76. Acosta-Urquidi, Juan, 2002, unpublished data.

77. Acosta-Urquidi, Juan, 2002, unpublished data.

Index

Page numbers in bold refer to photographs and figures; the letter t following a page number denotes a table.

153

Index

Index

Index

Index

Index

Printed in the United States
By Bookmasters